Intermittent Fasting Guide For Women Over 50

The Most Updated Guide to Losing Weight, Reset Your Metabolism, and Boost Your Energy.

100 Recipes and 28 Days Meal Plan Included

Amber Lane

Unlock a World of Books Before Anyone Else!

WE INVITE YOU TO JOIN OUR ELITE READERS' INNER CIRCLE!

As an elite reader, you will have the unique opportunity to access our preview books **for free**

(e.g. you could have read this book, in preview, for free)

SCAN THE QR CODE OR VISIT

wiseapublishing.com/innercircle/join

See you inside!

© Copyright 2021 Amber Lane - All rights reserved.

The content contained within this book may not be reproduced, duplicated, or transmitted without direct written permission from the author or the publisher.

Under no circumstances will any blame or legal responsibility be held against the publisher, or author, for any damages, reparation, or monetary loss due to the information contained within this book. Either directly or indirectly.

Legal Notice:

This book is copyright protected. This book is only for personal use. You cannot amend, distribute, sell, use, quote, or paraphrase any part, or the content within this book, without the author's or publisher's consent.

Disclaimer Notice:

Please note the information contained within this document is for educational and entertainment purposes only. All effort has been executed to present accurate, up-to-date, and reliable, complete information. No warranties of any kind are declared or implied. Readers acknowledge that the author does not render legal, financial, medical, or professional advice. The content within this book has been derived from various sources. Please consult a licensed professional before attempting any techniques outlined in this book.

By reading this document, the reader agrees that under no circumstances is the author responsible for any losses, direct or indirect, which are incurred as a result of the use of the information contained within this document, including, but not limited to, — errors, omissions, or inaccuracies.

Table of Contents

- INTRODUCTION 6
- INTERMITTENT FASTING: HOW IT WORKS 8
  - How Does It Work? 9
  - The Science Behind IF 10
- PROS AND CONS 11
  - Pros 11
  - Cons 12
- POSSIBLE NEGATIVE EFFECTS OF IF 13
- THE BODY CHANGES IN WOMEN OVER 50 15
  - What Happens to the Body of a Menopausal Woman? 15
  - The Ideal Diet for Menopause 16
  - Perimenopause 17
- WHY IF OVER 50? 18
- TYPES OF INTERMITTENT FASTING 20
  - Water Fasting 20
  - 16 and 8 21
  - 5:2 21
  - Eat-Stop-Eat 22
  - Alternate Day Fasting 22
  - Women-Specific Methods of Intermittent Fasting 23
  - Customizing IF for Postmenopausal Women involves several considerations: 24
- FIND OUT YOUR INTERMITTENT FASTING PLAN 25
- 12 MYTHS ABOUT IF TO DISPEL 29
- FOOD TO EAT AND TO AVOID DURING IF ... 33
  - What to Eat 33
  - What to Avoid 34
- PROVEN TIPS FOR MANAGING YOUR FAST ... 36
  - Don't Get Bored 36
- Zero-Calorie Beverages 36
- Don't Get Overwhelmed 36
- Have a Good Attitude 37
- Make Use of BCAAs 37
- Fast While You Sleep 37
- Use Proper Portion Control 37
- Closely Monitor Your Results 38
- MISTAKES TO AVOID 39
  - Switching Too Fast 39
  - Choosing the Wrong Plan for Your Lifestyle ...40
  - Eating Too Much or Not Enough 40
  - Your Food Choices Are Not Healthy Enough ...41
  - You Are Not Drinking Enough Fluids 42
  - You Are Giving Up Too Quickly 42
  - You Are Getting Too Intense or Pushing It ...43
- HOW TO DEAL WITH BAD DAYS WITH IF 44
  - It All Starts With Your Mindset 45
  - Adjust Your Priorities 46
  - Gravitate to Positivity 46
  - Rethink Punishments and Rewards 46
  - Identify "Troublesome Thoughts" 46
  - Don't Step On the Scale 46
  - Speak to Yourself as a Friend 46
  - Forget About the Entire "Foods" Attitude ..47
  - Focus On the Attainable 47
  - Envision a Better Life 47
  - Believe You Are in Control 47
  - Get to Learn How to Cope 48
  - Eliminate the Clutter and the Chaos 48
  - Concentrate on Solutions and Not Explanations 48
  - Say Thank You 48
  - Talk With Your Doctor 49
  - Other Changes in Lifestyle Which Promote Healthy Eating 49

BEST HOME EXERCISE DURING YOUR IF 51
- Weightlifting 51
- Pushups 51
- Running/Treadmill 52
- Squats 52
- Dips 52
- Reverse Lunge 52
- Planks 52
- Burpee 53
- Yoga 53
- Walking the Stairs 53

BEST APPS FOR YOUR IF 54
- Ate Food Journal 54
- BodyFast 54
- DoFasting 54
- FastHabit 55
- Fastic 55
- Fastient 55
- LIFE Intermittent Fast Tracker 55
- Simple 55
- Vora 55
- Window 55
- Zero 55

FAQ 56

BREAKFAST RECIPES 60
- 40-Second Omelet 60
- Mexican Egg & Veggie Skillet 60
- Stuffed Breakfast Veggie Cups 61
- Cheesesteak Quiche 61
- Homemade Low-Carb Muesli 61
- Low-Carb Egg Sandwich 61
- Southern Style Cauliflower Grits 62
- Almond & Berry Overnight "No-Oats" 62
- Spicy Almond Mix 62
- Low-Carb Burritos with Eggs and Mexican Sausage 62

VEGETABLE RECIPES 63
- Italian Eggplant Salad 63
- Mix Berry Coleslaw 63
- Roasted tomatillo salsa 64
- Smoothie bowl 64
- Vegan shortbread cookies 64
- Crepes with blueberries 65
- Festive Cranberry Stuffing 65
- Simple Puerto Rican sofrito 65
- Broccoli blossom 65
- Coconut curry cauliflower 66

POULTRY RECIPES 67
- Chicken Veronique 67
- Cauliflower-Rice Pilaf 67
- Chicken Salad 68
- Turkey Salad 68
- Curry Chicken 68
- Easy Chicken and Pasta Dinner 69
- Chicken Waldorf salad 69
- Salisbury Steak 69
- Basic Chicken Loaf 69
- Stir Fry Meal 70
- Fajitas 70

SEAFOOD AND FISH RECIPES 71
- Grilled Trout 71
- Baked Salmon 71
- Coconut Fish Dream 72
- Broiled Garlic Shrimp 72
- Shrimp Fajitas 72
- Spanish Paella 73
- Shrimp Salad 73
- Seafood Croquettes 73
- Salmon Salad 74
- Crab Cakes 74

SALAD RECIPES 75
- Crunchy Cauliflower Salad 75
- Buttermilk Herb Ranch Dressing 75
- Green Beans Salad 76
- Violet, Green Salad 76
- Cabbage with Strawberries 77
- Creamy Fruit Salad 77
- Broccoli Rice Salad 77

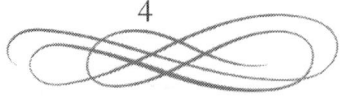

- SHRIMP SALAD WITH CUCUMBER MINT 78
- FIRE AND ICE WATERMELON SALSA 78
- RICED CAULIFLOWER SALAD 78
- FRUITY CHICKEN SALAD 78
- LEMON CURRY CHICKEN SALAD 79

SNACKS & SIDE RECIPES 80
- ANYTIME ENERGY BARS 80
- EASY BAKED PEARS 80
- SUNSHINE CARROTS 81
- SOUTHERN-FRIED OKRA 81
- CHAMP – SIDE DISH CAULIFLOWER MASH 81
- SLOVAKIAN SAUERKRAUT AND ZUCCHINI NOODLES 81
- DEVILED EGGS 82
- TACO SEASONING 82
- SWISS CHARD CROSTINI 82
- SPICED PEPITAS 82

MEAT RECIPES 83
- BEEF CURRY 83
- BEEF CASSEROLE 83
- HAWAIIAN-STYLE SLOW-COOKED BEEF 84
- FIESTA LIME TACOS 84
- SEASONED PORK CHOPS 84
- PARSLEY BURGER 84
- EASY BEEF BURGERS 85
- TORTILLA BEEF ROLLUPS 85
- JAMAICAN BEEF PATTIES 85
- CHILI RICE WITH BEEF 86

SOUP & STEW RECIPES 87
- THAI CHICKEN SOUP 87
- CAULIFLOWER RICE SOUP 87
- MINESTRONE SOUP 88
- QUICK MUSHROOM BROTH 88
- CHICKEN AND CORN CHOWDER 88
- SIMPLE SOUP BASE 89
- TEXAS-STYLE CHILI 89
- VIBRANT CARROT SOUP 89
- GREEN BREAKFAST SOUP 89
- VEGETABLE STEW 90

DRINK & BEVERAGE RECIPES 91
- APPLE CUP CIDER 91
- MIXED BERRY PROTEIN SMOOTHIE 91
- LEMON-STRAWBERRY PUNCH 91
- VEGAN HOT CHOCOLATE 92
- MEXICAN COCONUT DRINK 92
- LEMONADE 92
- FRUITY BAKED TEA 92
- STRAWBERRY SESAME MILKSHAKE 93
- RHUBARB TEA 93
- GREEN KIWI SMOOTHIE 93

DESSERT RECIPES 94
- SUGARLESS PECAN AND RAISIN COOKIES 94
- CRISPY BUTTERSCOTCH COOKIES 94
- EASY SPICY ANGEL CAKE 95
- APPLE FILLED CREPES 95
- CHOCOLATE COVERED STRAWBERRIES 95
- APPLE OAT SHAKE 96
- MOLTEN MINT CHOCOLATE BROWNIES 96
- BLUEBERRY WHIPPED PIE 96
- YELLOW CAKE 96
- TROPICAL FRUIT SALAD WITH BASIL LIME SYRUP 97

CONVERSION CHART 98

28-DAYS MEAL PLAN 99

A FREE GIFT FOR YOU 102

CONCLUSION 103

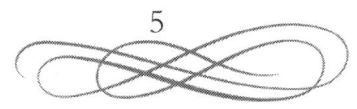

Introduction

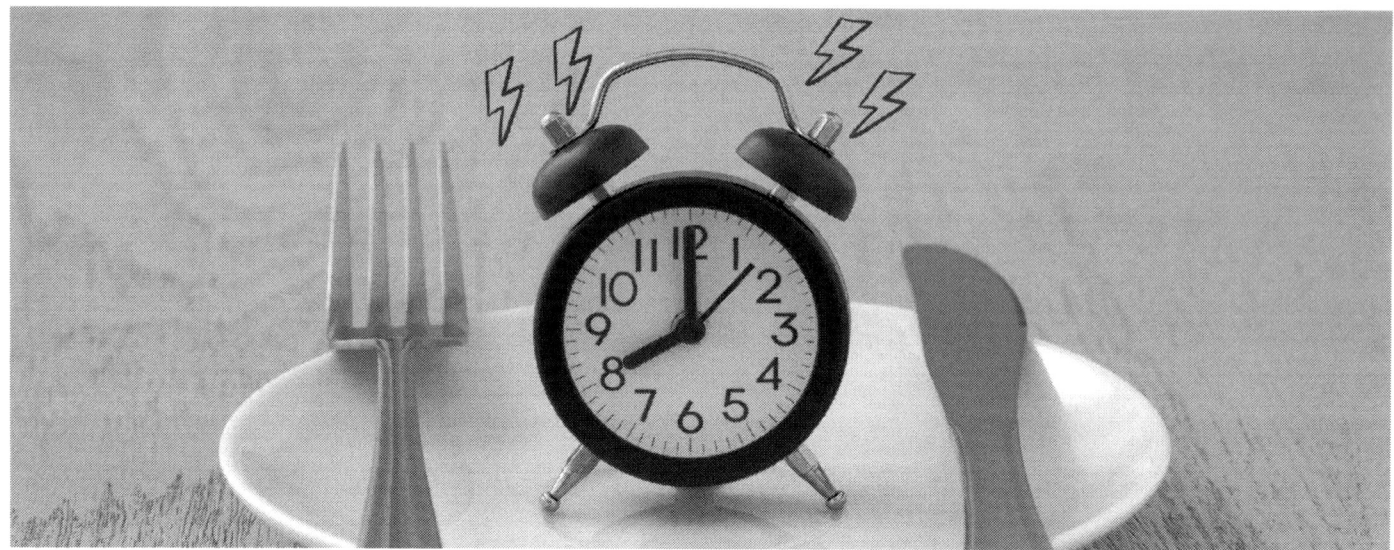

There are so many strategies for losing weight. How do you know where to start? **Women have different needs than men** regarding diet, exercise, and weight loss, and it seems that many popular strategies are aimed at men who want to look like muscular bodybuilders. Many of these programs leave you hungry and unsatisfied, leading to quitting early without seeing results.

Intermittent Fasting (IF) is a natural way to make you feel and look better in your 50s. Your body was designed to eat this way and has been confused by the never-ending availability of food and snacks. This form of patterned eating will restore your energy levels, retain your needed body muscle while reducing body fat, and improve your overall health and wellness. The major problem with traditional diets is that they are just hard to stick to. You deny yourself your favorite food and snacks in hopes of weight loss, and when you slip up, you feel ashamed and guilty, derailing your entire routine.

Cycling your eating pattern through periods of eating and fasting is as natural to your body as breathing. Humans have been eating this way for thousands of years, and only recently have we muddled our hunger signals so significantly that they are working against us instead of for us. Allowing yourself unrestricted access to food and snacks daily alters your body's chemistry, increasing the production of hunger-signaling hormones. These hormones now tell your body constantly that you are hungry, and they are hard to ignore! Intermittent Fasting will reprogram these hormones, decreasing your hunger signals and resigning them to the proper times of the day.

Changing the way you eat is also difficult. **You are setting yourself up for failure by denying**

yourself your favorite meals. Intermittent Fasting allows you to enjoy your favorite foods, snacks, and drinks as long as you consume them within your non-fasting window. Limiting the time you have available to consume calories will restrict the total number of calories you'll ultimately consume, providing weight loss with little effort. Fasting for weight loss differs from a religious fast or fasting before a medical procedure. It does not mean you don't eat anything and wait for the pounds to fall off. You simply limit your total caloric intake during specific periods (hours of the day or days of the week, depending on which method of Intermittent Fasting you feel is most appropriate for you) while enjoying a normal diet and lifestyle the rest of the time! Reducing the amount of food you eat for short periods is simpler and easier to stick to for most women, resulting in success and dedication without throwing in the towel.

The longer you practice Intermittent Fasting cycles, the easier you'll find them. Your body will adjust, you'll feel more motivation and energy, and you'll wonder how you could have eaten the food you used to all day! **This guide will explain in simple terms the science behind Intermittent Fasting, the benefits you can expect, and how to implement the plan into your life.**

Intermittent Fasting: How It Works

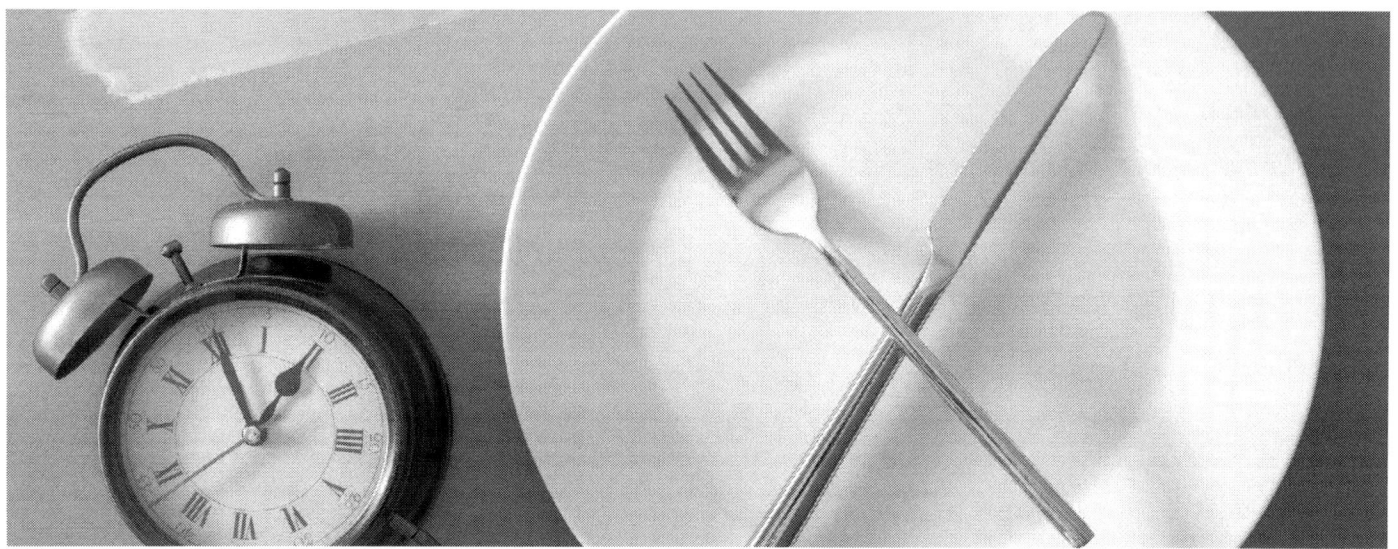

Basically, fasting is defined as abstaining from eating anything. It is the deliberate action of depriving the body of food for more than six hours. Intermittent Fasting is one of its forms; the fast is carried out cyclically to reduce the overall caloric intake in a day. To most people, it may sound unhealthy and damaging for the body, but **scientific research has proven that fasting can produce positive results on the human mind and body**. It teaches self-discipline and fights against bad eating practices. It is an umbrella term used to define all voluntary forms of fasting. This dietary approach does not restrict the consumption of certain food items; rather, **it reduces the overall food intake**, leaving enough space to meet the body's essential nutrients. Therefore, it is far more effective and much easier to implement, given that the dieter completely understands the nature and science of Intermittent Fasting.

Intermittent Fasting is categorized into three broad food abstinence methods: **alternate-day fasting, daily restrictions, and periodic fasting**. The means may vary, but the end goal of Intermittent Fasting remains the same: achieving a better metabolism, healthy body weight, and an active lifestyle. The American Heart Association, AHA, has also studied Intermittent Fasting and its results. According to the AHA, **it can help counter insulin resistance and cardiometabolic diseases, leading to weight loss.** However, a question mark remains on the sustainability of this health-effective method. The 2019 research "Effects of Intermittent Fasting on Health, Aging and Disease" has also found Intermittent Fasting to be effective against insulin resistance, inflammation, hypertension, obesity, and dyslipidemia. However, the work on this dietary approach is still underway, and the traditional methods of fasting, which existed for almost the entire human history in every religion from Buddhism to Jainism, Orthodox Christianity, Hinduism, and Islam, are studied to found relevance in today's age of science and technology.

How Does It Work?

Intermittent Fasting works between alternating periods of eating and fasting. It is a much more flexible approach, as there are many options to choose from according to body type, size, weight goals, and nutritional needs. The human body works like a synchronized machine that requires sufficient time for self-healing and repair. Constantly eating junk and unhealthy food without considering our caloric needs leads to obesity and toxic build-up in the body. That is why fasting is a natural means of detoxifying the body and providing enough time to utilize fat deposits.

Whatever the human body consumes is ultimately broken into glucose, which is later utilized by the cells in glycolysis to release energy. As the blood glucose level rises, insulin lowers the levels, allowing the liver to carry out De Novo Lipogenesis. The excess glucose is turned into glycogen and ultimately stored into fat, resulting in obesity. Intermittent Fasting seems to reverse this process by deliberately creating energy deprivation, which is then fulfilled by breaking down the existing fat deposits.

Intermittent Fasting works through lipolysis; though it is a natural body process, it can only be initiated when the blood glucose levels drop to a sufficiently low point. That point can be achieved through fasting and exercising. When a person cuts off the external glucose supply for several hours, the body switches to lipolysis. Breaking the fats also releases other by-products like ketones, which can reduce the body's oxidative stress and help detoxify.

Mark Mattson, a neuroscientist from the Johns Hopkins Medicine University, has studied Intermittent Fasting for almost 25 years of his career. He laid out the workings of Intermittent Fasting by clarifying its clinical application and the science behind it. According to him, Intermittent Fasting should be chosen as a healthy lifestyle.

While discussing the application of this dietary approach, it is imperative to understand how Intermittent Fasting stands out from everyday dieting practices. It is not mere abstinence from eating. What is eaten in this lifestyle is equally important as fasting itself. It does not result in malnutrition but promotes healthy eating and fast food. Intermittent Fasting is divided into two different states that follow one another. The cycle starts with the "Fed" state, followed by a "Fasting" state. The duration of the fasting state and the frequency of the fed state are established by the method of Intermittent Fasting. High

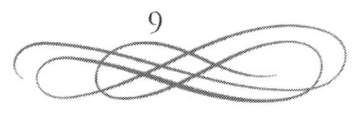

blood glucose levels characterize the latter, whereas, during fasting, the body gradually declines glucose levels. This decline in glucose signals the pancreas and the brain to meet the body's energy needs by processing the available fat molecules. However, if the fasting state is followed by a fed state in which a person binge eats food rich in carbs and fats, it will be more hazardous for their health. Therefore, the fasting period must be accompanied by a healthy diet.

The Science Behind IF

Biologically, Intermittent Fasting works at many levels, from cellular to gene expression and body growth. It is important to learn about the role of insulin levels, human growth hormones, cellular repair, and gene expression to understand the science behind the functioning of Intermittent Fasting. Intermittent Fasting firstly lowers glucose levels, which in turn drops insulin levels. This insulin lowering helps burn fat in the body, thus gradually curbing obesity and related disorders. Controlled levels of insulin are also responsible for preventing diabetes and insulin resistance. On the other hand, Intermittent Fasting boosts the production of human growth hormones up to five times. The increased production of HGH aids in quick fat-burning and muscle formation.

During the fasting state, the body goes into the process of self-healing at cellular levels, thus removing unwanted, non-functional cells and debris. It creates a cleansing effect that directly or indirectly nourishes the body and allows it to grow under reduced oxidative stress. Likewise, fasting even affects gene expression within the human body. The cell functions according to the coding and decoding of the gene's expression; when this transcription occurs at a normal pace in a healthy environment, it automatically translates into the longevity of the cells, and fasting ensures unhindered transcription. Thus, Intermittent Fasting fights aging and cancer and boosts the immune system by strengthening the body's cells.

Pros and Cons

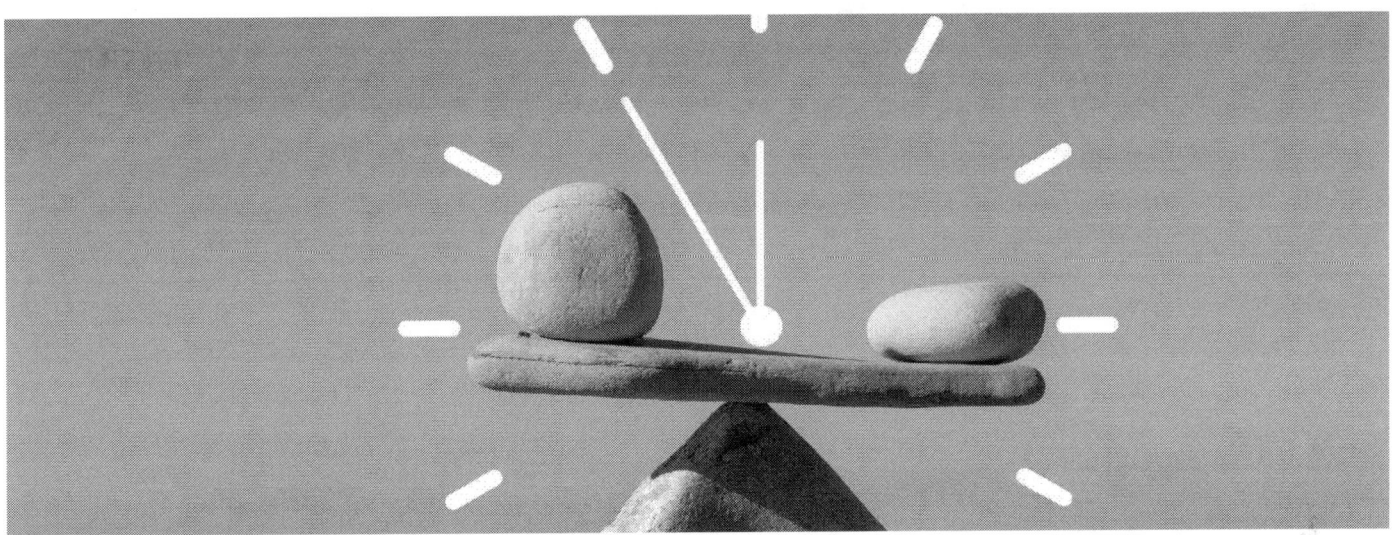

The different dietary examples have gotten consideration as an approach to reach and maintain a solid weight and pick up well-being benefits even in healthy people.

Research is progressing to understand the upsides and downsides of Intermittent Fasting completely. Long-term studies aim to know if this eating style gives enduring advantages.

Pros

Simple to Follow

- **Key Advantage**: No complex food rules; simply eat during designated times based on your chosen IF protocol.
- **Implementation**: Requires just a watch or calendar to track fasting and eating periods.

No Need for Calorie Counting

- **Benefit**: Avoids the tedious task of tracking every calorie, making weight management less burdensome.
- **How it Works**: Natural calorie reduction occurs due to limited eating windows, facilitating weight loss without meticulous counting.

Freedom from Macronutrient Restrictions

- **Flexibility**: No need to limit carbs, fats, or proteins, offering a less restrictive dietary approach.
- **Simplicity**: No specific cooking skills or dietary overhauls needed, just regular eating during non-fasting periods.

Unrestricted Eating

- **Enjoyment**: Allows for indulgence in favorite foods during non-fasting times, potentially reducing overall intake while still enjoying a variety of foods.
- **Psychological Benefit**: May ease the mental challenge of dieting by eliminating the feeling of constant deprivation.

Might Boost Longevity

- **Animal Insights**: Research on rats shows calorie restriction during fasting boosts lifespan and reduces disease rates, notably cancer.
- **Human Potential**: Enthusiasts believe these benefits also apply to humans, though conclusive long-term studies are still needed.
- **Research Backing**: Observational studies hint at fasting's role in extending life, but pinpointing the exact cause remains challenging.

Shedding Pounds Effortlessly

- **Proven Results**: 2018 research review reveals significant fat loss in clinical trial participants, independent of BMI.
- **Comparison with Traditional Diets**: Studies suggest intermittent fasting's weight loss efficiency parallels that of constant calorie restriction, with effectiveness possibly varying by age.

Glucose Control

- **Diabetes Management**: Some experts argue intermittent fasting can aid those with type 2 diabetes in controlling glucose levels, though findings are mixed.
- **Recent Studies**: A 2019 study observed that HbA1c levels rose over two years in both intermittent fasting and continuous calorie restriction groups, suggesting potential challenges in long-term glucose management.
- **Ongoing Debate**: While intermittent fasting may offer some advantages over constant calorie restriction for managing HbA1c levels, further research is necessary to solidify these findings.

Cons

Possible Side Effects

- **Common Issues**: Mood swings, tiredness, and headaches can occur, especially during the initial adjustment to fasting periods.
- **Medication Interactions**: Fasting may complicate timing for medication that needs to be taken with food.

Decreased Physical Activity

- **Observation**: Some individuals may experience decreased energy, impacting their ability to maintain regular exercise routines.

Challenges with Hunger and Overeating

- **Hunger**: Fasting periods can intensify feelings of hunger, especially in social settings.
- **Overeating Risk**: Unrestricted eating during non-fasting periods may lead to overindulgence, counteracting the benefits of fasting.

Lack of Nutritional Guidance

- **Nutrition**: IF focuses on timing rather than food quality, potentially neglecting the importance of a balanced, nutritious diet.

Long-Term Limitations

- **Research Gaps**: Long-term effects and safety of IF are still under investigation, highlighting the need for medical guidance when adopting IF.

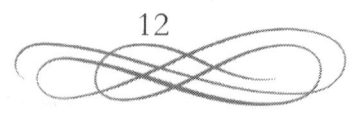

Possible Negative Effects of IF

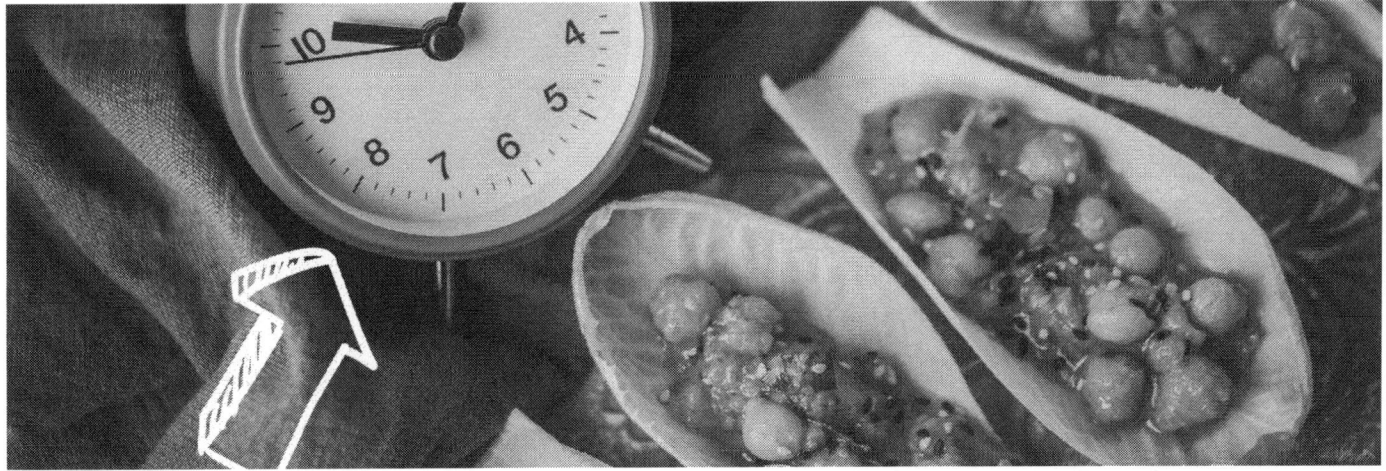

Intermittent fasting can benefit health but poses specific risks for women over 50, due to menopausal hormonal changes affecting blood sugar and hormones. It's essential to tailor IF approaches carefully for their safety and effectiveness.

Anxiety Attacks: Understanding and Managing Your Concerns

- **Why It Happens**: Skipping meals can trigger anxiety attacks, especially for those new to intermittent fasting or during menopause due to hormonal changes.
- **How to Ease Into It**: Start with a gentler fasting approach, like the 12-hour fast, to help your body adjust without overwhelming it.

Digestive Distress : Finding Your Balance

- **Detoxing Effects**: Initial fasting may lead to digestive changes as your body clears out toxins.
- **When to Worry**: Severe diarrhea warrants a doctor's visit. Moderate symptoms are typically part of the adjustment process.

Blood Sugar Levels: Keeping Them Steady

- **Individual Variations**: Some may find maintaining stable blood sugar levels challenging during fasting.
- **Strategies for Success**: Gradually transition into fasting, focus on nutrient-rich foods, and engage in light activities like walking or yoga.

Hormonal Imbalances: Navigating the Changes

- **Possible Disruptions**: Headaches, fatigue, and menstrual irregularities might signal a hormonal imbalance.
- **Solution**: Pause fasting if you experience these signs and consult your doctor for advice on nutritional adjustments.

Headaches: Staying Hydrated and Relaxed

- **Common Causes**: Low blood sugar and dehydration can lead to headaches.
- **Prevention Tips**: Drink plenty of water and manage stress to help prevent headaches during fasting.

Cravings: Managing Your Desires

- **Understanding Cravings**: Fasting can intensify cravings, especially for sweets or carbs.
- **How to Cope**: Balance your diet with complex carbohydrates and healthy fats to manage cravings and maintain energy.

Energy and Mood Adjusting

- **Early Challenges**: You may experience energy dips and mood swings as your body adapts.
- **Adapting Strategies**: Moderate your activity levels and practice mindfulness to support your body's transition.

Excess Urination: Keeping Hydrated

- **Why It Happens**: Increased liquid intake during fasting leads to more frequent bathroom visits.
- **Staying Hydrated**: Drink water regularly to prevent dehydration, regardless of increased urination.

Digestive Changes: Managing Heartburn, Bloating, and Constipation

- **Adjustment Period**: Your digestive system may need time to adapt to new eating patterns.
- **Balancing Your Diet**: Include fiber and protein-rich foods to ease digestive changes and stay hydrated to reduce discomfort.

Feeling Cold: A Sign of Change

- **Body's Adjustment**: Increased blood flow to fat stores for energy can make extremities feel colder.
- **Understanding the Shift**: This is a natural response as your body becomes more efficient at burning fat.

Overeating: Avoiding the Pitfall

- **Temptation After Fasting**: The urge to overeat when breaking a fast is common but counterproductive.
- **Mindful Eating**: Practice controlled, mindful eating to avoid undoing the benefits of fasting.

Hunger Pangs: Listening to Your Body

- **Feeling Hungrier**: It's normal to feel hungrier when adjusting to fasting schedules.
- **Dealing With Hunger**: If hunger becomes too distracting, consider adjusting your fasting window or plan nutrient-dense meals to enhance satiety.

The Body Changes in Women Over 50

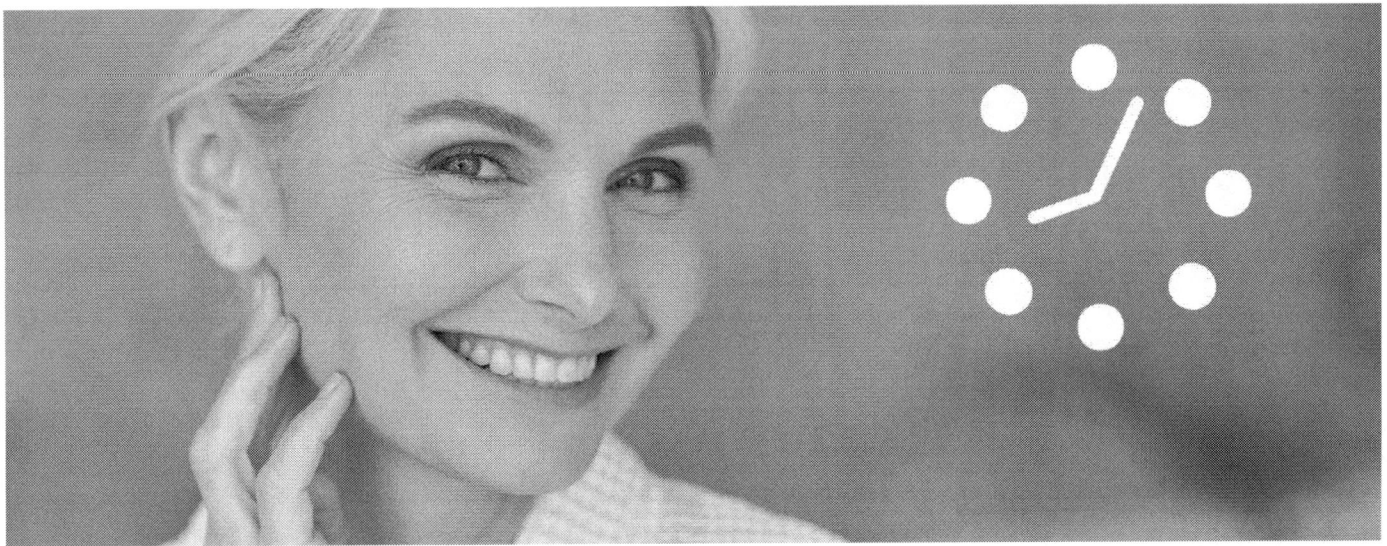

Menopause is one of the most difficult phases in a woman's life. It's a time when our bodies begin to change, and important natural transitions occur that are too often negatively affected, while it is important to learn how to change our eating habits and patterns appropriately. It often happens that a woman is not ready for this new condition and experiences it with a feeling of defeat as an inevitable sign of time passing, and this feeling of prostration turns out to be too invasive and involves many aspects of one's stomach.

It is therefore important to remain calm as soon as there are messages about the first signs of change in our human body, to ward off the beginning of menopause for the right purpose, and to minimize the negative effects of suffering, especially in the early days. Even during this difficult transition, targeted nutrition can be very beneficial.

What Happens to the Body of a Menopausal Woman?

It must be said that a balanced diet has been carried out in life, and there are no major weight fluctuations; this will no doubt be a factor that supports women who are going through menopause, but it is not a sufficient condition to present with classic symptoms that are felt, which can be classified according to the period experienced. We can distinguish between the pre-menopausal phase, which lasts around 45 to 50 years and is physiologically compatible with a drastic reduction in the production of the hormone estrogen (responsible for the menstrual cycle, which starts irregularly). Complex and highly subjective endocrine changes accompany this period. Compare effectively: headache, depression, anxiety, and sleep disorders.

When someone enters actual menopause, estrogen hormone production decreases even more dramatically, and the range of the symptoms widens, leading to large amounts of the hormone, for example, to a certain class called catecholamine adrenaline. The result of these changes is a dangerous heat wave, increased sweating, and the presence of tachycardia, which can be more or less severe.

However, the changes also affect the female genital organs, with the volume of the breasts, uterus, and ovaries decreasing. The mucous membranes become less active, and vaginal dryness increases. There may also be changes in bone balance, with decreased calcium intake and increased mobilization at the expense of the skeletal system. Because of this, there is a lack of continuous bone formation, and conversely, erosion begins, predisposing to osteoporosis.

Although menopause causes major changes that greatly change a woman's body and soul, metabolism is one of the worst. During menopause, the absorption and accumulation of sugars and triglycerides change. Increasing some clinical values , such as cholesterol and triglycerides, is easy, leading to high blood pressure or arteriosclerosis. In addition, many women often complain of disturbing circulatory disorders and local edema, especially in the stomach. It also makes weight gain easier, even though you haven't changed your eating habits.

The Ideal Diet for Menopause

Navigating menopause requires a strategic yet flexible approach to your diet, a period marked by significant changes that demand attention and care. With estrogen levels on the decline, the body's nutritional needs shift, impacting everything from bone density to how fat is distributed around your body. This stage can introduce new challenges, emphasizing the importance of adapting your diet to meet these changing needs effectively.

Menopause signals the need for increased nutrients such as calcium for bone health, while a slower metabolism and changes in fat distribution call for a careful review of your eating habits. Incorporating a balanced diet becomes crucial, blending a mix of nutrient-dense foods to support overall health and mitigate menopausal symptoms.

Reducing intake of high-carbohydrate foods can help manage insulin levels and maintain stable blood sugar, a key factor in navigating the metabolic changes during menopause. Equally, focusing on quality protein sources and healthy fats can support your body's needs during this time. Integrating foods rich in phytoestrogens, like soy and flaxseeds, can offer natural support for hormonal balance, while antioxidants from berries, nuts, and green tea protect against oxidative stress.

Digestive health may also take a hit during menopause, with changes in intestinal function leading to discomfort. A diet rich in fiber from fruits, vegetables, and whole grains can aid digestive health and help manage weight by keeping you fuller for longer. Omega-3 fatty acids, found in fish, walnuts, and flaxseeds, are essential for heart health, especially important as the risk of cardiovascular issues can increase post-menopause.

For bone health, key during this life stage due to the increased risk of osteoporosis, calcium and vitamin D are vital. Dairy products, leafy greens, and fortified foods can help meet these nutritional needs, ensuring your body remains strong and resilient.

Menopause is a call to fine-tune your diet, paying close attention to your body's signals and adjusting your food intake to support your health and well-being during this transformative phase. This personalized approach allows for a smoother transition, ensuring that you can embrace menopause not just as a challenge, but as an opportunity for positive change.

Perimenopause

There are many ways to lose weight during perimenopause, such as intuitive eating, a low-carb diet, a ketogenic diet, and more. If you are experiencing menopausal symptoms along with an unhealthy lifestyle (i.e., high intake of carbs, sugar, or processed foods), then you may need help in other areas as well (exercising regularly) before choosing an approach. Trying several approaches may be ideal for your body and life stage.

Understanding your perimenopausal symptoms will help you determine which dietary approach and exercise regimen is best for you. If you find any of the following signs, then these should be your first concern:

- Aging or weight gain.
- Significant mood swings or depression.
- Low libido, hot flashes, night sweats, or difficulty sleeping.
- Difficulty concentrating, memory loss, impatience, and irritability.
- Constantly tired or needing caffeine after lunch to wake up in the afternoon.

These are not all signs associated with perimenopause; there are many others.

Why IF Over 50?

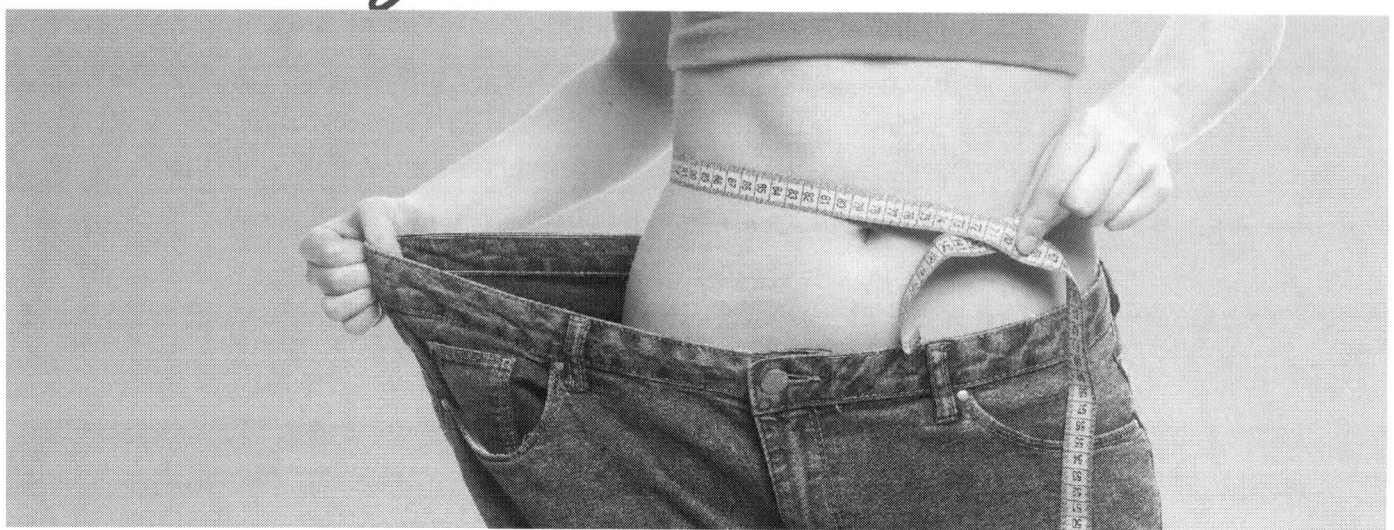

Expanding on the benefits and applications of intermittent fasting (IF) for women over 50, we delve deeper into how this dietary strategy specifically addresses the health challenges faced by this demographic. IF offers a strategic approach to mitigate these risks and improve overall health by addressing the root causes and contributing factors of these conditions.

Hypertension: Finding Balance with IF

- **The Issue**: Blood vessels lose elasticity with age, leading to hypertension, affecting two-thirds of women in this age group.
- **IF Solution**: Weight loss through IF eases cardiovascular stress, promoting healthier blood pressure.

Diabetes: A Proactive Approach

- **Rising Concerns**: Declining insulin sensitivity increases type 2 diabetes risks, especially post-menopause.
- **IF's Role**: Enhances insulin action, addressing the root cause and offer a proactive approach to maintain optimal health, manage weight, and reduce the likelihood of diabetes and its associated health issues.

Heart Health: Protecting Your Lifeline

- **Plaque Formation**: Excessive eating leads to heart disease, affecting many women aged 40 to 58.
- **IF Benefits**: Improves lipid profiles, reducing arteriosclerosis and heart disease risks.

Obesity: A Weighty Issue

- **Beyond Extra Pounds**: Obesity's link to over 20 chronic diseases highlights the need for effective management.
- **IF's Strategy**: Supports weight management, addressing obesity's health impacts.

Arthritis: Easing the Burden

- **Joint Wear and Tear**: Arthritis, exacerbated by excess weight and aging, limits mobility.
- **IF's Relief**: Reduces body fat and inflammation, alleviating arthritis symptoms.

Osteoporosis: Strengthening Bones

- **A Fragile Framework**: Over 53.9 million Americans face the risk of osteoporosis and fractures.
- **IF's Support**: Promotes bone density through diet and weight management, lowering fracture risks.

Cancers and Tumor: A Preventative Measure

- **Cellular Clean-Up**: Autophagy, triggered by IF, removes damaged cells, aiding in cancer prevention.
- **Lifestyle Choices**: Fasting reduces cancer risk, emphasizing the role of diet and exercise.

Menopause: Smoothing the Transition

- **Symptom Management**: Hot flashes, mood swings, and sleep disturbances mark this phase.
- **IF's Advantage**: Addresses belly fat and reduces the risk of metabolic and cardiovascular diseases.

Tailoring IF to Your Lifestyle

For women over 50, incorporating IF requires a personalized approach, taking into account health status, nutritional needs, and physical capacity. Consulting healthcare professionals can ensure that IF supports overall well-being without compromising joint health or nutritional balance. This customized approach underscores IF's versatility as a health-enhancing tool during a critical period of transition.

Types of Intermittent Fasting

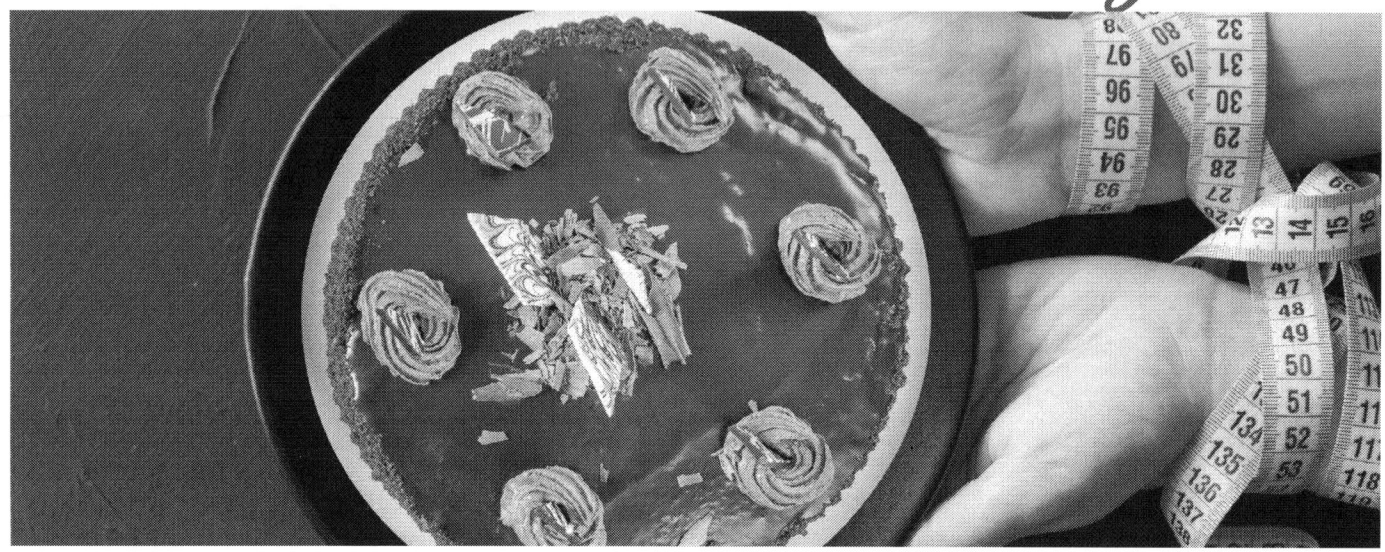

You must upregulate its functioning within your cells to harness and manipulate autophagy to benefit your body. There are various ways to do this, and we will look at them and how they work so that you can better understand how they affect your body. By upregulating autophagy, you can make your body resistant to many diseases.

Water Fasting

Dive into the transformative world of water fasting, an ancient yet powerful method that goes beyond mere weight loss to offer deep cellular rejuvenation. Imagine giving your body nothing but pure water for up to 72 hours—a cleanse so profound, it's like hitting the reset button on your health. While the idea might seem daunting, with medical guidance, water fasting can unlock a world of benefits.

Ever been told to fast before a medical procedure? That's water fasting in action—a sneak peek into its power to prepare your body for healing. But it's not just about pre-surgery prep; many embrace water fasting as a deliberate strategy to detoxify, launching the body into a state of autophagy. This remarkable process is nature's way of spring cleaning, where your cells discard the old and damaged, paving the way for fresh, vibrant cells. Imagine reducing your risk of diseases like cancer and Alzheimer's, not to mention potentially adding years to your life, all through the cleansing magic of fasting.

But the benefits don't stop with autophagy. Water fasting can be a gateway to lower blood pressure, improved cholesterol levels, and enhanced insulin function, leading to better blood sugar control. Yet, it's not a journey to embark on lightly. Safety first—consulting with a healthcare provider is non-negotiable to ensure your fasting path is both safe and suited to your body's needs. For women navigating the complexities of post-menopause, caution and moderation are key, with shorter fasts recommended to safeguard energy and metabolic health.

Embarking on a water fast isn't just about the fast itself; it's a holistic ritual of preparation and mindfulness. Gradually reducing your food intake before your fast can make the transition smoother, minimizing shock to your system and aligning your body with the rhythm of fasting. And while the scale might show a quick drop in weight, remember, true health transformation goes beyond just shedding pounds—it's about giving your body a foundation for long-term wellness.

As you step into the world of water fasting, remember to listen to your body, hydrate meticulously, and approach your fasting journey with flexibility and care. This isn't just a diet trend; it's an opportunity to reconnect with the innate wisdom of your body and embrace a healthier, more vibrant you.

16 and 8

In this method, you would eat for 8 hours of the day and fast for 16 hours. When doing this method of IF, you would usually skip breakfast and eat between 1 pm and 9 pm or 12 noon and 8 pm. The hours you choose can vary depending on your work schedule and lifestyle, but the key is that you eat for 8 hours and have a longer portion of the day in which you are fasting. It is the most popular method of IF and is the easiest if you are new to following specific diets. Many people will naturally eat during an 8-hour window of the day if they do not tend to eat breakfast, which is why this method is the easiest to transition to. Some people prefer to use different ranges of hours, but in terms of research, 16 and 8 be the most effective. If you are looking for something a little different, we will look at the two next most common methods below.

5:2

This method is different from the other two in that it involves some calories instead of hours. However, similar to the previous method, you are breaking up your week into different days instead of breaking up your day into hours.

In this method, you will restrict your caloric intake to between 500 and 600 calories on two days of the week. It is similar to the Eat-Stop-Eat method, except that you will greatly restrict your caloric intake instead of fully fasting on Monday and Thursday (for example). You will eat as you normally would for the other five days of the week. It is a method of intermittent eating, though it does not involve complete fasting. This method would be good for those who cannot completely fast for two days a week but want to try a form of intermittent eating still. For example, this would

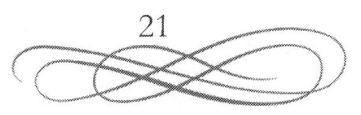

be a good option for someone who works a physically laborious job and cannot feel light-headed during the workday.

But specially this method allows for some flexibility and can be less intensive, making it suitable for those concerned about energy dips and hormonal imbalances.

Eat-Stop-Eat

This method is a little different than the 16 and 8 methods, as instead of breaking the day into hours, you would be breaking your week into days. You would fast for either one or two days of the week, not on back-to-back days. For example, you would fast from after lunch on Monday until after lunch on Tuesday and again beginning after lunch on Thursday. You could normally eat as you wish for all the other days of the week. This type is similar to water fasting in that it is a period where you are fasting, which is 24 hours long. However, it is intermittent, lasts only 24 hours, and repeats twice weekly. Water fast could be a one-off for 72 hours.

With this method, you must remember that what you choose to eat and in what quantities on the days you are not fasting will affect the results you see. You want to ensure you are not bingeing on the days you are not fasting. This method is a good choice for those who prefer more flexibility during their eating times and do not want to restrict their eating to a small 8-hour window, namely those who want to eat breakfast. It could be good for those with long working days and who prefer to have a longer time to eat during the day.

This approach demands caution. For postmenopausal women, ensuring nutrient-dense food intake during non-fasting days is crucial to support overall health.

Alternate Day Fasting

This fasting method involves fasting every other day and eating normally on non-fasting days. Like other forms of IF, you can drink as much as you want calorie-free drinks such as black coffee, tea, and water. You would fast for 24 hours on your fasting days, from before dinner one day to before dinner the next. Depending on the person, this method can be very successful or unsuccessful. The problem with this plan is that it can lead to bingeing on non-fasting days. If you do not tend to binge, you may enjoy the flexibility this diet offers by allowing you to eat whatever you want on alternating days.

There is a modification that some people choose to apply to this form of IF, where they allow themselves to eat 500 calories on their fasting days. It works out to about 20-25% of an adult person's daily energy needs, which will still put you in an extreme calorie deficit for those days, leading to the induction of autophagy. This method allows a person to continue with this diet consistently for longer than they may be able to with full fasts. It has the same effectiveness and works better with our modern lifestyles.

This type of IF is very beneficial for weight loss and is a good choice for those with such a goal as their main priority. Because of the calorie deficit, it puts a person; they are using energy than they are putting into their body, which leads to a breakdown of fat stores and weight loss.

Women-Specific Methods of Intermittent Fasting

Some evidence suggests that Intermittent Fasting affects men's and women's bodies differently. Women's bodies are much more sensitive to small-calorie changes, especially small negative variations in the intake of calories. Since women's bodies are made for conceiving and growing babies, women must be sensitive to modifications that may occur in the body's internal environment to a larger degree than the bodies of men to ensure that they will produce healthy and strong progeny. For this reason, some women may have trouble practicing Intermittent Fasting according to the above methods.

These methods may involve too much restriction on a woman's body, and she may feel some negative effects such as light-headedness or fatigue. To prevent this, some adjusted methods of Intermittent Fasting will work better for women's bodies. It is not to say that women cannot practice IF or fasting of any sort, but that they must keep this in mind when trying a fasting diet. Women can take a modified approach to fast so that the internal environment of their bodies remains healthy. Some slightly different patterns of IF may be safer and more beneficial for women. We will look at these below.

Crescendo

This method is quite similar to the Eat-Stop-Eat method, except that the hours have been changed slightly in this one. This fasting regimen involves breaking up the week into days and the days into hours. In this case, the woman should fast for 14 to 16 hours twice a week and normally eat every other day. These fasting days would not be back-to-back and would not be more than twice per week.

Alternate Day 5:2

Alternatively, she could fast every other day but only for 12-14 hours, eating normally on the days in between. On the fasting days, she would eat 25% of her normal calorie intake, making it a reduction in calories and not a full-blown fast.

14 and 10

In this method, the day would be broken up into hours. The woman would fast for 14 hours of the day and eat for 10 hours. Beginning with this modified version will allow her body to become used to fasting. Eventually, when comfortable, she can change the hours by one hour per day to reach 16 and 8.

By reducing the hours of the fast to 14 hours or less, women can still experience the benefits that IF can have for weight loss and autophagy induction without putting themselves in danger. It is not to say that women cannot fast in the same way that men can, but that they must start slowly and gradually increasing their hours of fasting so that they do not shock their bodies. When it comes to health, we must acknowledge that the bodies of men and women are built differently and, thus, will respond differently to changes.

12 and 12

Women can also benefit from reducing their fasting window to 12 hours. This method can be beneficial initially while your body gets used to fasting, and you can gradually work your way up from here. In this method, you would normally only eat three hours before you go to sleep, and then you could begin eating again early enough in the morning to have your first meal be breakfast. For example, if you go to bed at 10 pm, you only eat until 7 pm. Then you could eat breakfast after 7 am. It benefits people who like to eat breakfast and do not like to begin their day fasting.

For any person, regardless of their sex, the best approach to fasting may vary. When it comes to choosing an approach, being flexible is important. With dieting, the most important factor is consistency, so the best diet you can choose for yourself will be the one you can consistently maintain for a long time so that your body can adjust and changes can begin to occur.

Customizing IF for Postmenopausal Women involves several considerations:

Now let's look more specifically at personalizing IF for postmenopausal women:

- **Hydration**: Emphasizing hydration outside of fasting hours is essential, with a focus on drinking sufficient water and calorie-free beverages.
- **Modified Fasting Times**: Starting with a modified fasting approach, such as 14:10, can help ease into IF while monitoring energy and health responses.
- **Nutrient-Dense Foods**: Incorporating foods rich in calcium, vitamin D, magnesium, and omega-3 fatty acids during eating windows supports bone health, cardiovascular health, and hormonal balance.
- **Professional Guidance**: Consulting healthcare professionals before starting IF is crucial to tailor the fasting method to individual health needs and ensure safety.

By carefully adapting IF methods, postmenopausal women can enjoy the benefits of fasting, including potential weight loss and improved metabolic health, while minimizing risks. Listening to the body's signals and being willing to adjust the approach as needed are key to a successful fasting experience that supports well-being during and after menopause.

Find Out Your Intermittent Fasting Plan

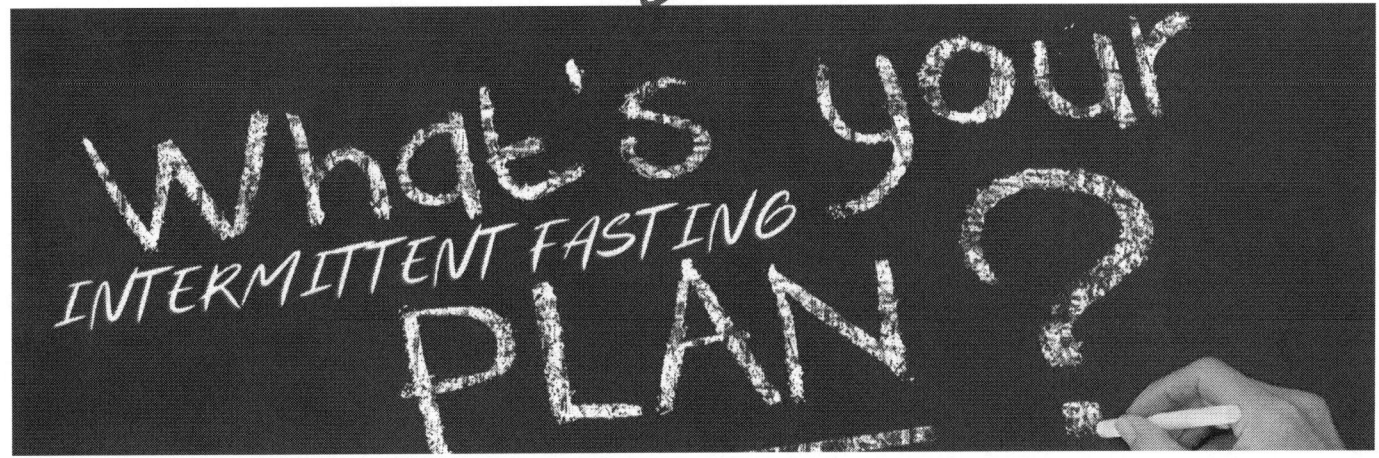

This section will help you understand exactly how to identify the best plan for an Intermittent Fasting program. Something to realize would be that the plan can be customized based on your needs. If you're trying to have eating schedules based on your lifestyle, chances are Intermittent Fasting is your solution. As you realize by now, there are many ways to follow Intermittent Fasting. We talked about the different Intermittent Fasting plans and which one will benefit you in what way. Remember that you will still see many benefits we discussed in the previous chapters, regardless of the plan you follow. It means that following Intermittent Fasting or a certain method should not demotivate you when following a certain plan.

Now that you know the different Intermittent Fasting methods available, it is time to select one. When choosing a method for yourself, keep in mind a few details. You must ask yourself several questions when choosing an Intermittent Fasting schedule. Below, I will show you the questions that will guide you in determining which method of Intermittent Fasting will fit best with your life.

1. What Does My Current Daily Schedule Look Like?

Take a look at your daily and weekly schedules. This action will give you insight into your busiest times of the day and when you will need energy the most.

2. When Am I Currently Fasting?

Everyone is fasting while they are sleeping. Do you normally wake up and wait to eat until lunch? Do you eat early in the morning but have a very small dinner? Any extended period without eating is considered a fast or even a mini fast. Pinpoint these times to incorporate a fasting schedule that will not disrupt your lifestyle too much. For example, if you usually skip breakfast and eat lunch around noon, you would have been fasting from when you last ate the night before until noon the next day (as long as you had nothing but water, black coffee, or black tea during that time). For this person, I would recommend a 16/8 or some variation of this, as they are already following something quite similar.

3. When Can I Not Afford to Fast?

Consider these when choosing your method if you have energy commitments, such as an after-dinner sports club or early morning meetings. You likely wouldn't want to skip dinner if you have evening commitments that require physical exertion. Likewise, eating breakfast first may be necessary to hit the ground running if you have morning meetings. If you have both of these, you may need to fast for 24 hours on the weekend when you have a less demanding schedule, as you need all the energy that food gives you throughout the week.

4. Can I Fast for 24 hours?

Not everyone can fast for 24 hours without some experience or an entire day put aside where they can relax while fasting. Can you put in the time and effort that a 24-hour fast requires, and can you deal with the side effects that could come with it, such as lethargy, irritability, headaches, and so on? If so, this method could work for you. If not, it is best to choose another.

5. What Are the Demands in My Life That May Cause Challenges?

Navigating the world of Intermittent Fasting (IF) can be a thrilling adventure, especially when life throws you curveballs like managing a bustling household, adhering to a rigorous exercise routine, or juggling a calendar filled with social commitments. The secret to mastering IF amidst this whirlwind? A dash of foresight, a sprinkle of strategy, and a generous portion of adaptability. Prepare to embrace the unexpected, ensuring you remain steadfast on your journey to wellness.

Dive deep into the essence of IF, where every question you ponder paves the way to a plan that resonates with the rhythm of your life. Whether it's the serene simplicity of the 16:8 approach, offering you hours of nourishment followed by rejuvenating fasting, or the tailored precision of the 5:2 method, where caloric mindfulness two days a week unveils a world of flexibility for the rest, discovering the right fit can transform your health narrative.

Remember, the path of IF is not set in stone. It's a journey of discovery, where the initial steps are merely the beginning. Should the winds of life steer you off course, fear not. The realm of IF is vast and varied, ready to accommodate your evolving needs with a simple tweak of timing or a bold leap into a new fasting style. This journey is as much about autophagy and the renewal it brings as it is about aligning with your body's whispers, urging you to pause, adjust, and proceed with renewed vigor.

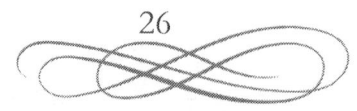

Within this dynamic landscape, you are the captain of your ship. While guides and maps—in the form of trainers and nutritionists—can offer valuable insights, the compass that truly guides you is your innate understanding of your body's needs and responses. Starting with an approach as accessible as the 16:8 method can open doors to a world where mental clarity and physical vitality become your steadfast companions, especially as you navigate the golden years beyond 50.

This adventure is not just about fasting; it's about crafting a lifestyle that embraces change, champions health, and celebrates every milestone along the way. So, gear up to explore the diverse methods of IF, each promising not just a transformation in body, but a rejuvenation of spirit and mind.

We will break down all the plans so you can better decide which one to pick and finalize.

16/8: As you know, the 16/8 method is one of the most popular methods for Intermittent Fasting. It will help you lose body fat but also help you with the anti-aging process and improve your overall function. Many people prefer this approach as it is the most convenient method to follow and is comfortably flexible. Depending on your lifestyle, this method could work very well when it comes to giving you the results that you're looking for.

This method's beauty is that you can build muscle, lose fat and do anything you want while making this a life choice. When I say a life choice, you can follow this plan for the rest of your life without feeling taxed. If feasible, we recommend that you follow the 16/8 method, one of the most studied ways of Intermittent Fasting.

12/12: This method is for someone looking to set up Intermittent Fasting without going too hard. If you don't know how Intermittent Fasting works or you don't know if it is going to be the right path for you, then you should start with the 12/12 method. This plan will allow you to get your feet wet when it comes to Intermittent Fasting so that you can continue with the program if you enjoy it or make it a bit more challenging by upping the fasting times.

That said, the 12/12 method is merely something to get your feet wet and not something you should do for the rest of your life. The secure troll's method is a great plan to start. However, except at the beginning, you will not see the anti-aging or weight loss effects you're looking for following this method. It is where the 16/8 method will shine, giving you enough time to fast while seeing the benefits you hope to get from Intermittent Fasting.

The water fast: The water fast is for someone looking to detoxify their body, but they're changing how their body functions. This plan is only to be followed to detoxify the gut so we can digest better. As you might know, the stomach is the second brain because your body heavily depends on your gut and how it digests. Eating food is necessary for living, so we must care for the organs, especially our gut. Make sure you use this method to clean out your organs and see better results. It will allow you to be in a better position when digesting food and keeping your organs beautiful and safe.

5:2 Diet: This fasting protocol is ideal for losing weight quickly. Now, if you are in this group and have the motivation and willpower to complete it, then the 5/2 works the best. This plan makes you lose much body fat quickly, allowing you to live much better overall.

Remember that following the 5/2 diet will not help you with any long-term anti-aging process. But I will help you detoxify your body and lose a ton of weight, especially in the beginning. Don't follow this protocol for the rest of your life, as it is not sustainable. However, once you get the hang of this plan, you will be much better positioned to lose fat and get your goal weight quicker than you would. Once you've practiced the 5/2 diet, we recommend following the 16/8 diet quickly. The 16/8 diet is where you want to be when it comes to see long-lasting results. Nonetheless, a 5/2 diet will work for you if you do a labor job, because of its structure.

Keep in mind that we want you to use your brain when it comes to picking out the right plan. As always, make sure that you know your body before you start following any of these programs. We recommend a start off with a 12/12 method as you will see significant benefits from it initially. However, once you get your feet wet with Intermittent Fasting, then we recommend that you start following other plans that will help you achieve that goal as well.

In light of the varied intermittent fasting (IF) methodologies discussed, I wish to emphasize essential principles to ensure your journey is both healthy and fruitful. It's crucial to attentively observe your body's reactions, making necessary adjustments to your fasting regimen should you experience heightened fatigue or emotional fluctuations. Recognizing and responding to your body's feedback allows for the customization of your fasting schedule, ensuring it complements periods of heightened activity and meets your energy demands, in harmony with your body's innate cycles.

Health must always take precedence over rigid adherence to fasting schedules. Adopt a adaptable stance, never overlooking the significance of staying hydrated and regularly seeking advice from healthcare experts well-versed in menopausal health. These professionals can offer tailored guidance, ensuring your IF strategy aligns with your overarching wellness objectives.

Establishing a community of support is also pivotal. Engaging with fellow women navigating fasting during this life phase can offer invaluable perspectives and moral support. The act of sharing insights and advice can prove to be a profound source of encouragement.

Customizing IF for women over 50 means tuning into and honoring your body's signals. By vigilantly tracking your reactions and judiciously implementing modifications, you can harness the advantages of IF while gracefully navigating the nuances of this life stage.

12 Myths About IF to Dispel

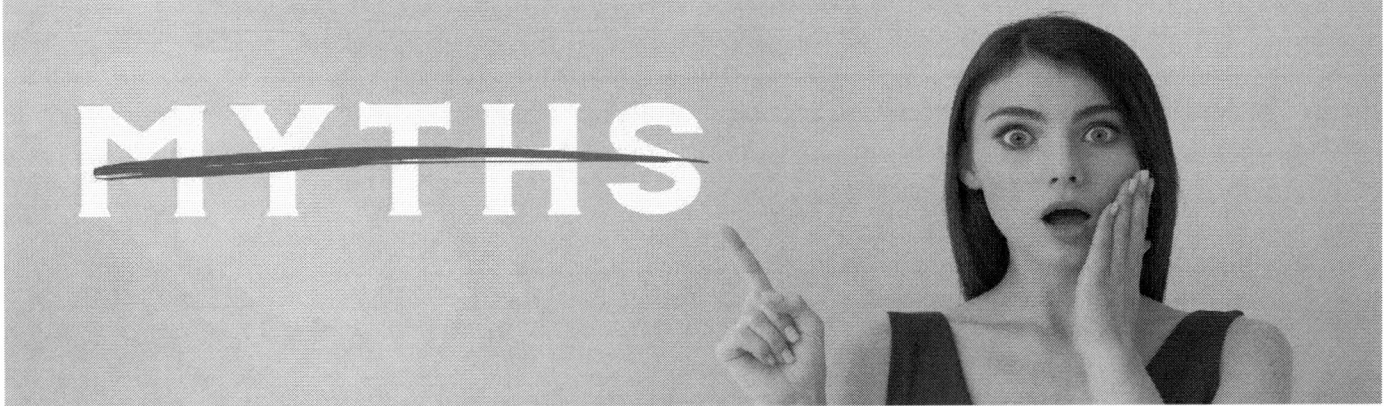

Issues that are not popular, such as Intermittent Fasting, can be misunderstood with many misconceptions and myths surrounding them. Many people with half-baked information suddenly become experts on the topic and are always willing to advise anyone ready to listen. It doesn't matter how long a false premise is considered correct; once the evidence is present, the error is exposed, and wise people will know to stick with the facts.

Myth #1: Intermittent Fasting Is Unsafe for Older Adults

Anyone can engage in Intermittent Fasting if they have no medical conditions and are not pregnant or lactating. Of course, our bodies do not all have the same tolerance levels, even in people who look identical. If one or more persons respond negatively to Intermittent Fasting because they are advanced in age and are women, it does not mean another will react the same way.

There is no doubt that Intermittent Fasting is not meant for everyone. Fasting is unsafe for children because they need all the food they can get for continual development. Fasting is not an issue for older people; any adult can fast.

Myth #2: You Gain Weight as You Age

A myth is a combination of facts and falsehood. It is a typical example of that. It says that growing older means your metabolism will slow down, and your body will not burn or use up calories as fast as when you were younger. However, weight gain in older adults is not an automatic fact. The key to keeping your body performing great is to develop and maintain healthy habits such as fasting intermittently, drinking enough water, reducing stress levels, and getting adequate exercise.

Myth #3: Your Metabolism Slows Down During Fasting

This myth represents one of those big misunderstandings I mentioned earlier. The difference between calorie restriction and deliberately choosing when to take in calories is huge. Intermittent Fasting does not necessarily limit calorie intake nor make you starve. When a person starves or undereats, changes occur in their metabolic rate. But there is no change whatsoever in your metabolism when you delay eating for a few hours by fasting intermittently.

Myth #4: You Will Get Fat if You Skip Breakfast

"Breakfast is the most important meal of the day!" It is one of the most popular urban myths about Intermittent Fasting. It is in the same category as the myths, "Santa doesn't give you presents if you are naughty" and "carrots give you night vision." Some people will readily point to a fat relative or friend because they don't eat breakfast. But the question is: are they fat because they don't eat breakfast or skip breakfast? After all, they are fat and want to reduce their calorie intake.

The best way to collect unbiased data when conducting scientific studies is through randomized controlled trials (RCTs). After a careful study of 13 different RCTs on the relationship between weight gain and eating or skipping breakfast, researchers from Melbourne, Australia, found that overweight and normal-weight participants who ate breakfast gained more weight than participants who skipped breakfast. The researchers also found a higher calorie consumption rate later in the day in participants who ate breakfast. It puts a hole in the popular notion that skipping breakfast will make people overeat later in the day (Harvard Medical School, 2019).

The truth is, there is nothing spectacular about eating breakfast as far as weight management is concerned. Limited scientific evidence disproves or supports the idea that breakfast influences weight. Instead, studies show no difference in weight loss or gain when one eats or skips breakfast.

Myth #5: Exercise Is Harmful to Older Adults, Especially While Fasting

No. It is not harmful to exercise while fasting. And no, exercise is not harmful to older adults, whether they are fasting or not. On the contrary, exercising during your fasting window helps to burn stored fats in the body. When you perform physical activities after eating, your body tries to burn off new calories that are ingested from your meal. But when you exercise on an empty or nearly empty stomach, your body burns fats stored already and keeps you fit.

What is harmful to older adults is not engaging in exercise at all. A lack of exercise or adequate physical activity in older adults is linked to diabetes, heart disease, and obesity, among other health conditions.

In a landmark study, researchers from Harvard Medical School demonstrated that frail and older women could regain functional loss through resistance exercise (Harvard Medical School,

2007). Participants from a nursing home (100 women aged between 72 and 98) performed resistance exercises three times a week for ten weeks. At the end of 10 weeks, the participants could walk faster and further, climb more stairs, and lift more weight than their inactive counterparts. Also, a 10-year study of healthy aging by researchers with the MacArthur Study of Aging in America found that older adults (people between 70 and 80) can get physically fit whether or not they have exercised at a younger age. The bottom line is as long as you can move the muscles in your body, do it because it is safe and will only help you live a better and longer life.

Myth #6: Frequently, Eating Reduces Hunger

There is mixed scientific evidence in this regard. Some studies frequently show that eating reduces hunger in some people. On the other hand, other studies show the exact opposite. Interestingly, at least one study shows no difference in the frequency of eating and how it influences hunger (US National Library of Medicine, 2013). Eating can help some people overcome cravings and excessive hunger, but there is no evidence to prove that it applies to everyone.

Myth #7: You Can't Teach an Old Dog New Tricks

The brain never stops learning nor stops developing at any age. New neural pathways are created when a person learns something new at any age. And with continued repetition, the neural pathways become stronger until the behavior is habitual. Older people are often more persistent and motivated than younger people when learning new things. Learning should be a lifelong pursuit, not an activity reserved for young people.

Don't allow anyone to convince you into believing that it is too late to learn new eating habits because you are in your golden years or are approaching it. It doesn't matter if you've never tried fasting; you can still train your brain to make fasting a habit even in old age. Start small, make it a natural occurrence in everyday life, repeating until you get used to it, and your positive results, like glowing skin and improved energy, will motivate you to make it into a lifestyle.

Myth #8: You Must Lose Weight During Intermittent Fasting

This myth is rooted in the hype that Intermittent Fasting has received in recent years. Unless done correctly, Intermittent Fasting may not yield weight loss benefits. To experience significant weight loss, you must eat healthily during your eating window. Equally, it is important to stick to the fasting schedule. If you keep cheating and adjusting your fasting window to favor more eating time, or you overeat during the eating window to compensate for lost meals, your chances of losing weight will greatly diminish.

Myth #9: Your Body Will Go into "Starvation Mode" If You Practice Intermittent Fasting

This myth is based on the misconception of starvation mode and what triggers it. First, starvation is when your body senses a significant drop in energy supply and reduces your metabolic rate. Simply put, it reduces the rate at which your body burns fat as a lack of food. It is an automatic response to conserve energy. It makes sense to reduce energy consumption if there is little to no supply of further energy from meals. In other words, if you stay away from food for too long, your body activates starvation mode and significantly stops further body fat loss.

Intermittent Fasting does not trigger starvation mode. Instead, it helps to increase your metabolic activities, meaning your body can burn more fat when you fast for short periods. Starvation mode is only triggered when you fast over 48 hours, a practice I do not recommend for older adults.

Myth #10: An Aging Skin is Better Taken Care of with Anti-Aging Cream

It is not necessarily true. Brown spots, sagging skin, and wrinkles can be reversed using expensive creams and topical treatments, especially if a dermatologist prescribes them. These topical products exfoliate the top layer of your skin and make them appear smoother. However, that result (clear, smooth skin) is only temporary.

Activating autophagy is a better way to look younger without any side effects. The way is to engage in mild stress-inducing activities, such as Intermittent Fasting and exercising. One key element to maintaining healthy skin is quenching your skin's thirst. Not drinking enough water can damage the skin, causing it to become dry and blemished, leading to wrinkles. Drinking adequate water is the best approach to successfully "take the years off" daily.

Myth #11: Fasting Deprives Your Brain of Adequate Dietary Glucose

Some people believe your brain will underperform if you don't eat carbohydrate-rich foods. This myth is rooted in the notion that your brain only uses glucose as fuel. But your brain doesn't use only dietary glucose for fuel. Some very low-carb diets can cause your body to produce ketone bodies from high-fat foods. Your brain can function well on ketone bodies. Continuous, Intermittent Fasting coupled with exercise can trigger the production of ketone bodies. Your body can also use a process known as gluconeogenesis to produce the sugar your brain needs. It means that your body can effectively produce it on its own without you feeding it with just carbs.

Intermittent Fasting does not interfere with brain function, fuel, or energy needs. However, because Intermittent Fasting is not suitable for everyone, if you feel shaky, dizzy, or extremely tired during fasting, consider talking with your doctor or reducing your fasting window.

Myth #12: Intermittent Fasting Will Make Older Adults Lose Their Muscle

First, considering older people as frail is stereotypical and largely incorrect. Frailty is not limited to just older adults and is a generalization of old age. Younger people can become frail if they suffer from a disabling chronic disease or have a poor diet. Scientists studied data from almost half a million people and found that middle-aged adults as young as 37 show signs of frailty (Mail Online, 2018).

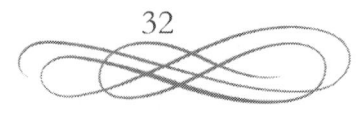

Food to Eat and to Avoid During IF

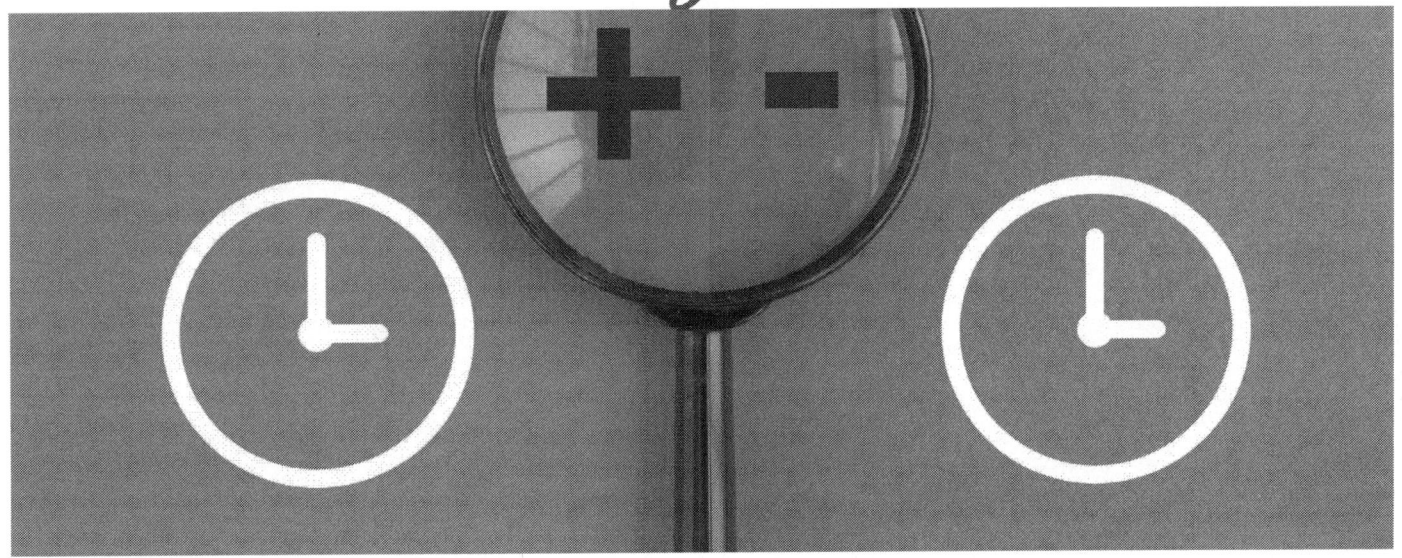

What to Eat

Berries
Berries are very healthy, incredibly flavorful, and much lower in calories and sugar than you might think! Their tart sweetness can bring a smoothie to life, and they make a delicious snack on their own without any help from things like cream or sugar.

Cruciferous Vegetables
These vegetables include cabbage, Brussels sprouts, broccoli, and cauliflower. These are wonderful additions to your diet because they're packed with vital nutrients and fiber that your body will love and use quickly!

Eggs
Eggs are a great addition to your diet because they're packed to the gills with protein; you can do almost anything with them. Eggs are easy to prepare, and they travel well if you hard boil them, and they can pair with just about anything. They're a great protein source for salads, and they're good on their own as well.

Fish
Fish is a wonderful source of protein and healthy fats. Whitefish, in particular, is typically very lean, but fish like salmon with a little color is packed with protein, fats, and oils that are great for you. They're good for brain and heart health; you can do many delicious dishes with them.

Healthy Starches Like Certain Potatoes (with Skins!)

Red potatoes, in particular, are perfectly fine to eat, even if you're trying to lose weight, because your body can use those carbs for fuel, and the skins are packed with minerals that your body will enjoy. A little bit of potato here and there can do good things for your nutrition, but they are also a great way to feel like you're getting a little more of those fun foods you should cut back on.

Legumes

Beans, beans, the magical fruit. They're packed with protein, and their starch makes them stick to your ribs without making you pay for it later. They're wonderful in soups, salads, and just about any other meal of the day that you're looking to fill out. By adding beans to your regimen, you might find that your meals stick with you a little longer and leave you feeling more satisfied than you thought possible.

Nuts

I know you've heard people talking about how a handful of almonds makes a great snack, and if you're anything like me, you've always had a hard time believing it. Nuts, as it turns out, have a good deal of healthy fats in them that your body can use to get through those rough patches, and while they are not the most satisfying snack on their own, you might consider topping your salad with them for a little bit of crunch or pairing them with some berries to make them a little more satisfying.

Probiotics to Help Boost Your Gut Health

Probiotics can be found in several ways in health food stores, but they can make digestion and gut health much more optimum. Often having a happy gut means your dietary success and overall health will improve!

Vegetables That Are Rich in Healthy Fats

Not to sound topical or trendy, but avocados are a great example of a vegetable packed with healthy fats. Look for vegetables with fatty acids and a higher fat content, and you will find that if you add more of those into your regimen, you will get hungry less often.

Water, Water, Water, and More Water

Stay hydrated no matter what you add to or subtract from your regimen. It will aid in digestive health and ease, keep you from feeling slumpy or tired, and keep you from getting too hungry. Add electrolytes where you need to, and don't be shy about bringing a bottle when you go from place to place. Stay hydrated!

What to Avoid

No food is strictly prohibited during Intermittent Fasting. However, some foods are less suitable for fast weight loss. In the recipes in this book, you will find some of these ingredients as well. It is not a problem to eat one of these foods now and then, knowing that they are more suitable during maintenance than during the slimming phase.

Grains

While grains may have health benefits and be full of fiber, you can also get these nutrients elsewhere. The human diet does not require grain consumption. While grains may have some benefits, they are ridiculously high in total and net carbohydrates. A single serving of brown rice contains 42 net carbs, almost double your net carb intake for an entire day.

Starchy Vegetables and Legumes

Some vegetables are high in carbohydrates. It includes potatoes, beets, corn, and more. These vegetables may have nutritional benefits, but you can get these nutrients in low-carb vegetable alternatives. To consider how high in carbs these options can be, a medium-sized white potato contains 43 net carbs (more than a serving of brown rice!), a standard sweet potato contains 23 net carbs, and a serving of black beans contains 25 net carbs.

Sugary Fruits

Most fruits have high sugar content, meaning they are also high in carbohydrates, which will spike your blood sugar and cause an insulin reaction. It is important to avoid most fruits to avoid this from happening. The exception is that you can enjoy berries, lemons, and limes in moderation. Some people will also enjoy a small serving of melon as a treat occasionally, but watch your portion size as it can add up quickly!

Milk and Low-Fat Dairy Products

Milk is much higher in carbohydrates than cheese, with a glass of two-percent milk containing 12 carbs, half your daily total. Instead, choose low-carb and dairy-free alternatives such as almond, coconut, and soy milk. You may consider using low-fat cheeses instead of full-fat to reduce the saturated fats you consume. But, if you want to reduce your saturated fat intake, choose lighter cuts of meat rather than low-fat dairy products. When the cheese is made with low-fat dairy, it naturally has a higher carbohydrate content, which will cut into your daily net carb total.

Cashews, Pistachios, and Chestnuts

While you can enjoy nuts and seeds in moderation, remember that nuts contain a moderate level of carbohydrates and, therefore, should be eaten in moderation. However, some nuts are high in carbs, and avoiding them, including cashews, pistachios, and chestnuts, is better.

If you want to enjoy nuts, instead of these options, you can fully enjoy almonds, pecans, walnuts, macadamia nuts, and other options.

Most Natural Sweeteners

While you can certainly enjoy sugar-free natural sweeteners such as stevia, monk fruit, and sugar alcohol, you should avoid natural sweeteners that contain sugar. Suffice it to say that sugar makes these sweeteners naturally high in carbs. Not only that, but they will also spike your blood sugar and insulin. Avoid honey, agave, maple, coconut palm sugar, and dates.

Alcohol

Alcohol is not generally enjoyed on any diet, as your body cannot burn off calories while your liver attempts to process alcohol. Alcohol adds unnecessary calories and carbohydrates to your diet. The worst offenders would be margaritas, piña coladas, sangrias, Bloody Marys, whiskey sours, cosmopolitans, and regular beers.

But, if you drink alcohol regardless, drink in moderation and choose low-carb versions, such as rum, vodka, tequila, whiskey, and gin. The next best options would be dry wines and light beers.

Proven Tips for Managing Your Fast

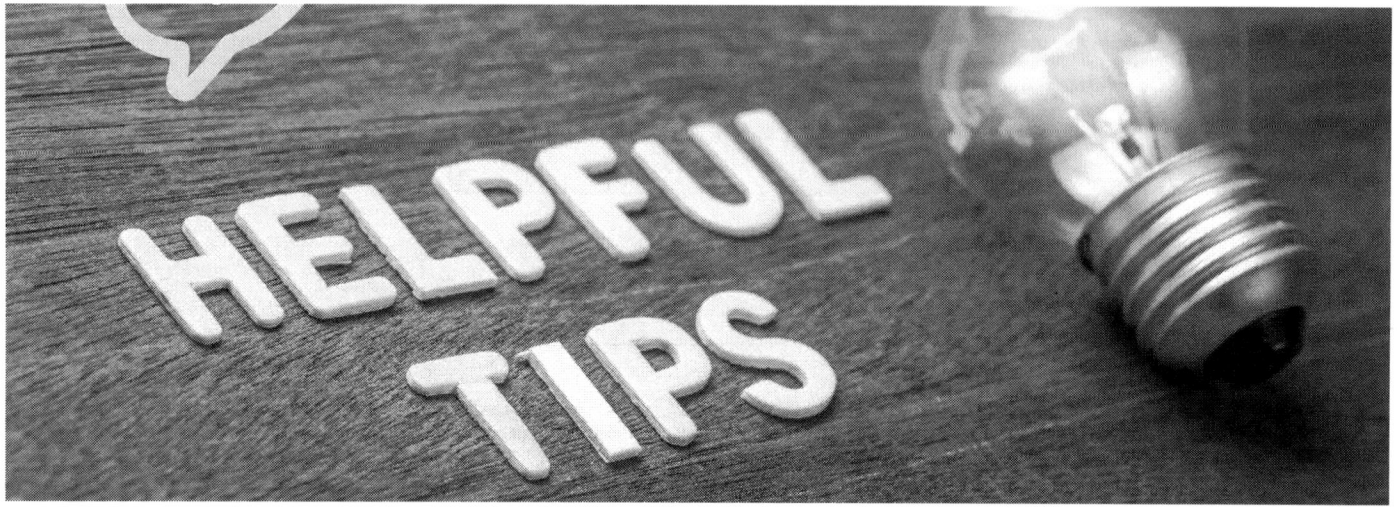

Intermittent Fasting doesn't have to be a struggle. If done right, it can be quite enjoyable, even life-changing. It's all just a matter of how you approach your fast. You must do what you can to make the best of it. In this chapter, we will review some tips and tricks to get you on the right path and ensure you succeed fast.

Don't Get Bored

One of the biggest pitfalls of Intermittent Fasting is boredom. Mindless eating, after all, often strikes because we don't have anything else to do. The more packed your itinerary is, the less likely you will succumb to eating out of sheer boredom. If you have a hobby, make full use of it. Blow off some steam with a pastime rather than mindlessly grazing through an afternoon. Just ensure that you don't get bored and will be more likely to stay on track.

Zero-Calorie Beverages

Simply drinking water or some other zero-calorie beverage can help temporarily fill you up and satisfy your appetite while you fast. Water, of course, is a good and filling zero-calorie beverage. It's nature's replenisher. But it's not the only one. Some good zero-calorie beverages include:

- Coffee (without cream or sugar)
- Springwater
- Tea (again, without cream or sugar)

Don't Get Overwhelmed

Many who start a regimen of Intermittent Fasting —especially if they have no previous experience with fasting— become a bit overwhelmed. Going into a fasting routine stressed out will only make things worse; however, whatever you do, make sure you don't stress out over your efforts. To avoid this, go into your Intermittent Fasting routine with the attitude that making mistakes is okay. If you slip up the first couple of times you fast, don't worry; correct yourself and try again. Intermittent Fasting, after all —in many ways— is a trial-and-error process. You must experiment and figure out exactly what works best for you, so give yourself enough breathing room.

Have a Good Attitude

It might seem like common sense in many ways, but it's worth saying regardless (attitude is everything). If you go into Intermittent Fasting with the attitude that you will fail, it probably won't be long before you conclude a self-fulfilled prophecy. On the other hand, if you take on a positive attitude of making the best of things, you will be that much closer to success. It's just as simple as that. And if you aren't in a good mood. Just fake it until you make it, and your spirits will begin to rise regardless.

Make Use of BCAAs

Just what are BCAAs, you might ask? That fancy little acronym stands for "Branch Chain Amino Acids," They are highly useful when it comes to girding your system for an intermittent fast. Among other things, BCAAs ensure you do not lose too much muscle while your body is burning up all that fat during a fast. Studies have shown that taking 10 g of a BCAA supplement before a fast can work wonders.

Fast While You Sleep

Unless you are engaged in an intermittent fast that takes up a whole 24-hour period, it's always advisable to situate most of your fast time during your sleeping hours. It means you could skip dinner or breakfast and sleep off the rest of your fast. If you want to fast for 16 hours, you could have an early evening meal at 5 pm and then not eat again until 9 am the next morning. It would complete a 16-hour fasting cycle without much feeling of deprivation. Just fast while you sleep, and your body will do the rest.

Use Proper Portion Control

When it comes to successful Intermittent Fasting, being able to use proper portion control is crucial. If your fast-day routine allows you to eat under 500 calories, portion control is necessary to keep yourself within your allotted limits. But perhaps even more importantly, it should be the portion control you exercise when it comes to your non-fast days, for it is the non-fast day that will have you tempted to go overboard and eat too much if you are not careful.

Intermittent Fasting, after all, recommends someone to fast, then normally eat, not fast, and then binge! Believe me! If someone starves themselves for 24 hours and then eats until they are stuffed the next day—they're not helping anyone! But there is a simple physiological reason that folks tend to get messed up regarding their portion control after a fast. You may notice that

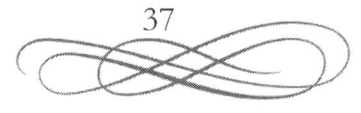

you cease to feel hungry after the first few hours of a fast.

Hunger pains are the body's built-in cue to eat. You may notice, however, that after the first few hours of a fast, your hunger subsides. It is because, by then, our body realizes that food is not forthcoming. For the rest of your fast, you may very well not feel all that hungry at all. But this is what happens, folks. After you end your fast and get out a bowl of pasta, the second you take that first bite, your body screams, "Oh wow, we have food now!"

And almost immediately, the hunger pains hit you with abandon, and your body is now working overtime to consume as much as you possibly can. It's just the way we are hardwired to be. Everything about the human condition is geared toward survival, and our ancestors in the past went through periods of feast and famine, often not knowing when the next meal would be. So our body will turn off the hunger signal when we do without for a while and poke, prod, and goad us into eating as much as possible when food is suddenly available.

That's great for someone who might not know when their next meal might be, but it's horrible for someone trying to plan an intermittent strategic fast under strict guidelines and protocol. That's why sometimes you might have to exercise a bit of mind over matter to keep yourself from overdoing it on your non-fast day, and proper portion control can be a real lifesaver when it comes to Intermittent Fasting.

Closely Monitor Your Results

For most of us, nothing serves to encourage us more than seeing good, positive results. And as you fast, monitoring your progress will help you improve problem areas and boost your self-confidence to show you how far you have come in the process. Also, as Intermittent Fasting is in many ways a trial-and-error process, tracking your journey in real-time enables you to tweak and finesse your experience until your methodology is optimal. Everyone is different, and Intermittent Fasting isn't a one-size-fits-all program. Monitoring your results will give you the feedback you need to improve when necessary and provide solid encouragement as you go.

Mistakes to Avoid

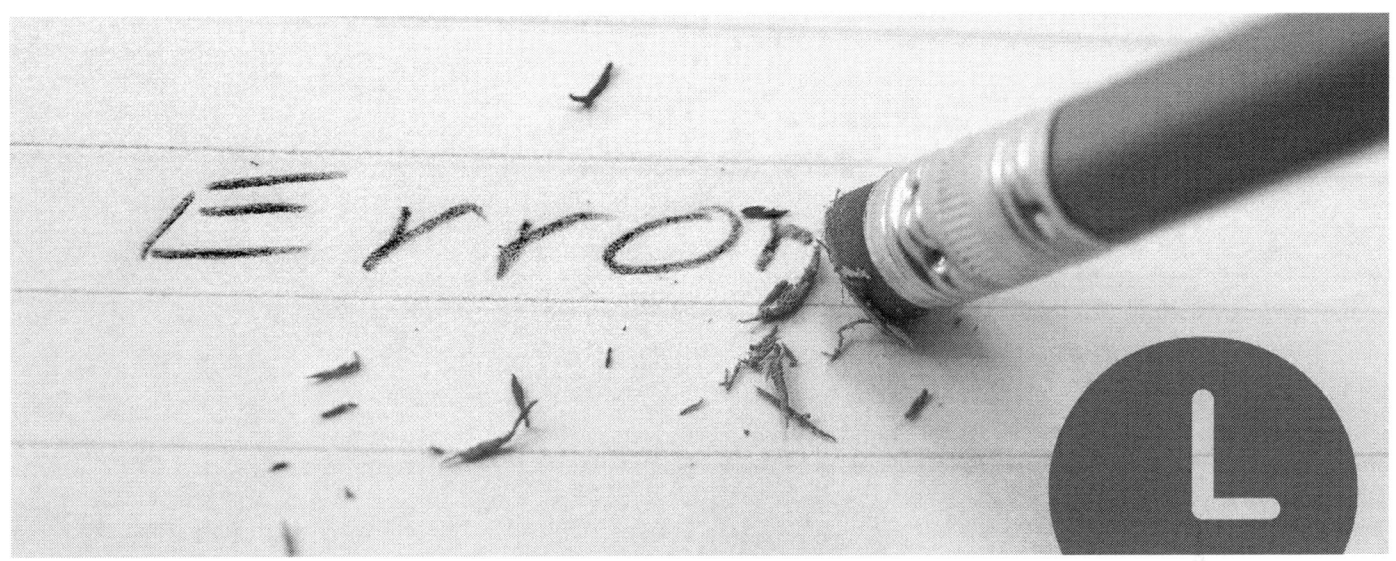

When you are looking to make significant adjustments in your life, it can take time to discover exactly how to do it in the best ways possible. Many people will make mistakes and have setbacks as they seek to improve their health through Intermittent Fasting. Some minor mistakes can easily be overcome, while others may be dangerous and cause serious repercussions if caught in time.

This chapter will explore common mistakes people make when on an Intermittent Fasting diet. We will also explore why these mistakes are made and how they can be avoided. You must read through this chapter before you commit to the diet itself. That way, you can ensure that you are avoiding any potential mistakes beforehand. It will help you avoid unwanted problems and achieve your results with greater success and fewer setbacks.

You should also keep this chapter handy as you embark on your Intermittent Fasting diet. That way, if you do begin to notice that things are not going as you had hoped, you can easily reflect on this chapter and get the information you need to adjust your diet and improve your results.

Switching Too Fast

A significant number of people fail to comply with their new diets because they attempt to go too hard too fast. Trying to jump too quickly can make you feel too extreme of a departure from your normal life. As a result, both psychologically and physically, you are put under significant stress from your new diet. This situation can lead to you feeling like the diet is ineffective and that you are suffering more than you benefit from it.

Switching to the Intermittent Fasting diet will take time and patience if you eat regularly and frequently snacks. I cannot stress the importance of your transition period enough.

It is common to want to jump off the deep end when making a lifestyle change. We often want to experience great results immediately and are excited about the switch. However, after a few days, it can feel stressful. Because you didn't give your mind and body enough time to adapt to the changes, you ditch your new diet in favor of more comfortable things.

Fasting should always be acclimated slowly; it might take some time. There is no set period; it must be done based on what feels right for you and your body. If you are not properly listening to your body and its needs, you will suffer in major ways. Especially with diets like Intermittent Fasting, letting yourself adapt to the changes and listening to your body's needs can ensure that you are not neglecting your body in favor of strictly following someone else's guide on what to do.

Choosing the Wrong Plan for Your Lifestyle

It is common to forget the importance of picking a fasting cycle that goes with your lifestyle and fitting it in. Trying to fast to a cycle that does not match your lifestyle will ultimately make you feel bothered by your diet and struggle to maintain it.

The way we naturally eat is often related to what we feel fits into our lifestyle in the best way possible. So, if you look at your present diet and notice that many convenience meals happen throughout the day, you can conclude two things: you are busy and eat when you can. Picking a diet that allows you to eat when you can is important in helping you stick to it. Similarly, you must search for healthier convenience options to get the most out of your diet.

Anytime you make a lifestyle change, such as with your diet, you must consider your lifestyle. You can completely adapt everything to suit your dreamy needs in an ideal world. However, in the real world, many aspects of your lifestyle are likely not practical to adjust. Picking a diet that suits your lifestyle rather than your diet makes far more sense.

Documenting your present eating habits before you embark on your Intermittent Fasting diet is a great way to begin. Focus on what you eat and how often, and consider diets that will serve your lifestyle. You should also consider your activity levels and how much food you need at certain times of the day. For example, fasting until noon might not be a good idea if you have a spin class every morning, as you could end up hungry and exhausted after your class. Choosing the dieting pattern that fits your lifestyle will help you maintain your diet to continue receiving great results.

Eating Too Much or Not Enough

Focusing on what you eat and how much you eat is important. It is one of the biggest reasons a gradual and intentional transition can be helpful. If you are used to eating throughout the day, attempting to eat the same amount in a shorter window can be challenging. You may feel stuffed and far too full of sustaining that amount of eating

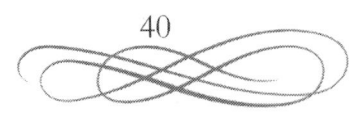

on a day-to-day basis. As a result, you may find yourself not eating enough.

If you are new to Intermittent Fasting and take the leap too quickly, it is common to find yourself scarfing down as much food as possible when your eating window opens again. As a result, you feel sick, too full, and uncomfortable. Your body also struggles to process and digest that much food after fasting for any given period. It can be even harder on your body if you have been using a more intense fast and then you stuff yourself. If you find yourself doing this, it may be a sign that you have transitioned too quickly and need to slow down and back off.

You might also find yourself not eating enough. Attempting to eat the same amount that you typically eat in 12-16 hours in just 8-12 hours can be challenging. It may not sound so drastic on paper, but if you are not hungry, you may simply not feel like eating. As a result, you may feel compelled to skip meals. It can lead to you not getting enough calories and nutrition daily. Ultimately, you are not eating enough and feeling unsatisfied during your fasting windows.

The best way to combat this is to begin practicing making calorie-dense foods before you start Intermittent Fasting. Learning which recipes you can make and how much food you need to help you reach your goals is a great way to get ready and show yourself what it truly takes to succeed. Then, begin gradually shortening your eating window and giving yourself the time to work up to ingest enough food during those eating windows without overeating. In the end, you will find yourself feeling amazing and not feeling unsatisfied or overeating as you maintain your diet.

Your Food Choices Are Not Healthy Enough

Diving into the world of diets like keto or trying your hand at Intermittent Fasting? Here's the scoop: it's not just about dodging the no-nos or picking the right eating window. The real game-changer is knowing the nuts and bolts of what your body craves nutrient-wise. Think of it as customizing your body's fuel mix for optimal performance. This means loading up on the right vitamins and minerals to keep your engine running smoothly.

Now, don't get it twisted. Intermittent Fasting isn't a free pass to indulge in a junk food bonanza within your eating windows. Spoiler alert: scarfing down bags of chips or cookies, even in the right time frames, won't do you any favors. The goal is to find a diet buddy that complements your fasting, whether it's the keto vibe, the Mediterranean flair, or another nutritious path. These aren't just diets; they're your roadmap to a nutrient-rich journey.

Choosing wisely is key to hitting those health goals. It's not just about losing weight; it's about fueling your body for a better hormonal balance and keeping the internal machinery in tip-top shape. That way, you're not just going through the motions; you're reaping the full spectrum of benefits and truly elevating your health game. So,

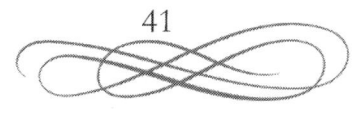

as you navigate through the fasting lanes, remember: it's what's on your plate that counts.

You Are Not Drinking Enough Fluids

Let's shake things up a bit! Did you know that munching on fruits and veggies not only fills you up but also sneaks a good dose of hydration into your day? It's like hitting two birds with one stone. But if your plate's been lacking in color lately, chances are you're not sipping enough H2O either. It's time to ramp up your hydration game!

Feeling groggy, crampy, or constantly hungry? You might just be dehydrated, especially if you're trying your hand at Intermittent Fasting. The fix? Keep water close—like, really close. Aim to take a gulp at least every 15 to 30 minutes. Trust me, it's a game-changer for flushing your system with the good stuff.

Don't just stop at water, though. Throw in some low-calorie sports drinks, bone broth, or even a cup of tea or coffee into the mix. These can be your hydration sidekicks, making sure you're not just hydrated, but also not bored out of your mind with plain water. Just watch those fasting calories; you don't want to mess with the fasting magic by going overboard.

If the desert starts creeping up on you (hello, dehydration symptoms!), up your water intake, stat. Letting dehydration go unchecked is like inviting a headache and muscle cramp party, and nobody wants an invite to that. And if you're the type who forgets to drink water, set a reminder. Your body will thank you.

How to know if you're nailing the hydration thing? Keep an eye on how often you're hitting the bathroom. Peeing at least once every hour? You're in the hydration sweet spot. If not, time to chug a bit more. Waiting until you're parched or aching to drink up is like waiting to run out of gas before filling up your car—it just doesn't make sense. Stay ahead of the game to keep your body thriving, not just surviving.

You Are Giving Up Too Quickly

Embarking on the Intermittent Fasting journey, many envision instant transformations, a swift shift towards their health goals. Yet, the reality of IF is more of a marathon than a sprint. Results, while often remarkable, don't materialize overnight. The timeline for witnessing the magic of IF is as diverse as our individual lives—shaped by how swiftly you adapt, the nature of your feasts within those precious eating windows, and the vigor of your daily activities.

It's easy to feel disheartened if the scale doesn't tip in your favor immediately or if the mirror doesn't yet reflect your aspirations. However, surrendering too soon is a disservice to your potential. Remember, for some, the fruits of their labor only become apparent after weeks of dedication. This delay doesn't spell failure; it's merely the time your body takes to calibrate, seeking the perfect equilibrium where health and satisfaction align.

Before you consider quitting, pause and reflect. A powerful tool at your disposal is revisiting your food diary. Spend a few days meticulously logging

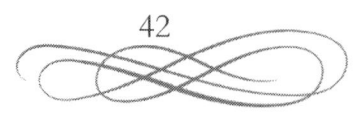

your meals and activities under the IF regime. This isn't just about what you eat but when and how your body responds to these choices, coupled with an honest assessment of your physical activity.

This introspective exercise often unveils that the absence of expected results may stem from an imbalance—perhaps an excess of indulgence or an underestimation of nourishment, relative to the energy you expend. Armed with these insights, adjusting your dietary approach becomes less about guesswork and more about strategic planning, paving the way for a regimen that truly resonates with your body's needs.

IF's efficacy isn't one-size-fits-all. Each of us carries unique nutritional needs and lifestyle factors that shape our journey. The commitment to discovering and fine-tuning the balance that works uniquely for you is the cornerstone of success in IF. With patience and perseverance, the rewards of your fasting endeavor are within reach, promising not just fleeting changes but a lasting transformation.

You Are Getting Too Intense or Pushing It

Chasing after your goals can sometimes lead you to push your limits, especially when it comes to dieting. You might find yourself trying out extreme fasting cycles or pushing your body beyond what it can handle in pursuit of those goals. However, going to such extremes often backfires rather than bringing you closer to your objectives. It's not just about reaching a goal; it's about doing so without compromising your well-being.

Remember, your body talks, and it's crucial to listen. Proper nutrition and exercise should enhance your health, not detract from it. Overdoing it can lead to serious, even life-threatening, consequences. Sure, pushing your limits is sometimes necessary, like when you're aiming to build muscle, but there's a fine line between effective exertion and harmful overexertion.

If your diet starts causing more harm than good, it's time to ease up. A few side effects might be normal at the start, but if they're severe, persistent, or returning, that's a red flag. Your aim should be to manage and reduce side effects, not to live with them permanently. After all, the whole point of adjusting your diet and lifestyle is to feel healthier, not worse.

Make it a habit to check in with yourself daily to ensure your physical needs are met. If something feels off or symptoms worsen, address them right away. Focusing on your long-term goals and understanding that health shouldn't be sacrificed for immediate results will not only help you achieve your goals but also leave you feeling better about your journey.

How to Deal With Bad Days With IF

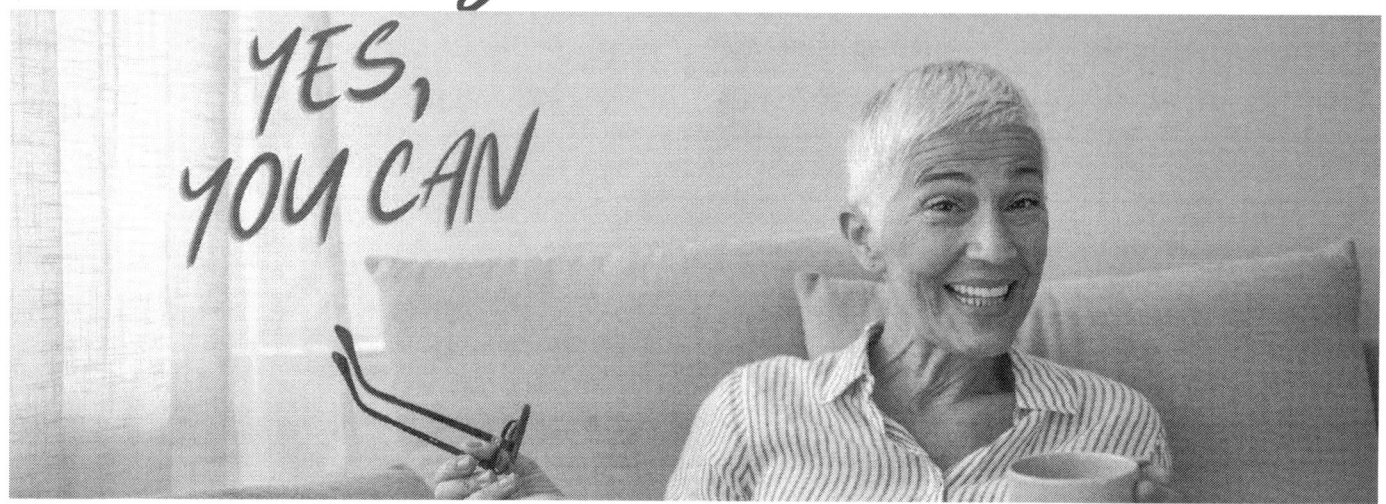

In today's world, we're bombarded with the message that eating right is the cornerstone of health, particularly for women over 50, who often hear that it's much easier to gain weight than to lose it. Despite the vibrant supermarket aisles, health posters, and TV ads promoting a healthy lifestyle, sticking to a nutritious diet remains a challenge. The problem isn't a lack of desire to eat healthily; it's often not knowing where to start or how to sustain these habits amidst our bustling lives.

Diving headfirst into a new diet often ends in frustration because many weight-loss plans feel like a square peg in a round hole compared to our everyday routines. Rather than chasing after temporary fixes, the goal should be to integrate lasting, meaningful changes into our diet. Success in maintaining healthy eating habits is achievable with realistic goals and perseverance, transforming what once seemed impossible into something entirely attainable.

Every diet has its pros and cons, but the real game-changer is shifting your mindset towards weight loss. Many approach dieting and exercise from a place of self-criticism, focusing on negative self-perceptions and quick fixes rather than the holistic benefits of better health, like improved well-being, a more vibrant life, and reduced risk of chronic diseases. This negative mindset can lead to disappointment and a cycle of unhealthy behaviors.

However, changing how you think about weight loss can make a profound difference. Research highlights the impact of our attitudes on our behaviors; for instance, feeling unhappy about one's body can deter exercise, and focusing solely on weight can paradoxically lead to weight gain. It's not just about psychology; even genetics and hormonal responses to stress, like cortisol secretion, can influence our weight.

In essence, embarking on a journey to better health requires more than just following a diet; it involves nurturing a positive mindset and recognizing that our self-view and attitude towards lifestyle changes are just as crucial as the food we eat.

It All Starts With Your Mindset

The hitch with the latest diet fads isn't their fancy meal plans—it's their failure to spark any real change in your thinking. They often demand sweeping changes to your diet, a strategy that's far from sustainable. The key to genuinely transforming your eating habits lies not in the food itself but in reshaping how you view food and health.

A common obstacle for those trying to eat better is what's known as a "closed mentality." This mindset traps individuals in the belief that change is impossible, leading them to embark on new diet plans with defeat already in mind. They might think their health woes are just bad genetics or fear that even attempting to address them would be too embarrassing or futile.

For those stuck in this mindset, any diet attempt might seem doomed from the start. They might even prefer their current state over the perceived stress of trying to change, believing it to be a safer, less challenging option. However, without a shift in mindset, the path to a healthier lifestyle is fraught with quick disappointment, since real change is a marathon, not a sprint. There are no miracle diets or secret foods, despite the hype you might read in magazines or see celebrities endorsing.

Enter the "growth mindset," a concept psychologists champion for its openness to change. Unlike the fixed mindset, which sees the status quo as unchangeable, the growth mindset embraces evolution and learning from mistakes. It understands that setbacks are just stepping stones towards bigger goals.

So, which mindset resonates with you? If you're leaning towards the fixed side, it's time to pivot towards growth. Start simple: gather information and keep a journal to track the gradual progress and the milestones you reach. This isn't about unrealistic goal-setting but about setting achievable targets and celebrating the small wins, like opting for healthier meals more frequently.

Recognizing that your mindset might be the barrier is a massive leap towards overcoming it. The great news? Acknowledging this is your first step towards meaningful change. Here are some practical tips to shift towards a growth mindset: maintain a journal, set realistic goals, and gradually increase your intake of nutritious meals. Remember, the journey to a healthier you is as much about changing your mind as it is about changing your diet.

Adjust Your Priorities

The reason might be to lose weight, but that should not be the target. Instead, the objectives should be small, manageable stuff you have full power to control. Have you consumed five fruit and veggie servings today? That's one goal achieved. What about 8 hours of sleep; have you got them in? If so, you can cross them off your list.

Gravitate to Positivity

It is vital to surround yourself with the good. Doing so offers a relaxing, socially healthy environment to invest in yourself. Don't be afraid to ask for help or support.

Rethink Punishments and Rewards

Remember that making healthier decisions is a way to practice self-care. Food is not a reward, and a workout is not a penalty. They are necessary to care for your body and make you do your best. You deserve both.

Taking a few minutes at the start of your exercise or the beginning of your day to calm down and simply concentrate on breathing will help you set your goals, communicate with your body, and even reduce your body's stress response.

Find a quiet space wherever you are (even at work) and try this exercise to help you feel more relaxed and ready to tackle the rest of your day. Lie with your legs outstretched on your back, and put one hand on your stomach and one on your shoulder. Breathe in for 4 seconds through your nose, stay for two, and exhale for six seconds through your mouth. Repeat this process for 5-10 minutes, focusing on the sensation of your stomach rising and falling with each breath.

Identify "Troublesome Thoughts"

Identify the feelings that bring you problems and seek to prevent and change them. Let them stop intentionally by saying "no" out loud. It may sound silly, but that simple action breaks your thought chain and helps you introduce a new, safer one. The easiest way to do so is to count as many times as you like, from one to 100, until your negative thoughts disappear.

Don't Step On the Scale

Even though stepping on the scale to check your progress is not bad, many people often associate it with negative thoughts. If you know the number on the scale will lead to negative and self-destructive thoughts, you should avoid it until you are in a place where the scale doesn't affect your mental health.

Speak to Yourself as a Friend

Regarding beauty and body image expectations, we're incredibly harsh on ourselves. We punish ourselves with the standard we set. It is a widespread problem for people today, especially women, with advertisements and images of a specific body type. Building a positive body image is an excellent way to counteract this negative stream of images to which we are encouraged to compare ourselves. Improving your body image can be hard, but it's certainly doable. Focus on your positive qualities, skills, and talents. Focus on appreciating and respecting what your body can

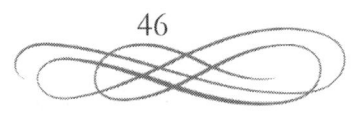

do. Say positive statements to yourself every day. Avoid negative or berating self-talk. Admire the beauty of others, but avoid comparing yourself to anyone else. Handle yourself like this.

Forget About the Entire "Foods" Attitude

We've learned somewhere along the way to feel either proud or bad for any food choice we make. But in the end, it's just food, so you shouldn't feel bad for enjoying an occasional cookie. Allow yourself to sometimes have a piece of chocolate cake or a glass of wine.

Treating yourself to some comfort food is right for your mind and body. It is doing it every day that sabotages weight loss. During a more or less strict diet, having a day in a week to get away from it is the key to success, the guarantee for motivation, and does not undermine the goal of losing weight.

Focus On the Attainable

If you've never been to a gym before, your goal on the day shouldn't be to do 30 minutes on the elliptical. Going for a 30-minute walk might be a better goal. If you want to cook more, but have little familiarity with healthier cooking, don't bank on creating new nutritious recipes every night after work. Instead, consider using a subscription service such as Blue Apron or HelloFresh, where pre-portioned recipes and ingredients are delivered to your doorstep, helping you learn different components, make new meals, and develop your cooking skills.

Envision a Better Life

What will life be like if you put good habits in place? Will you be more comfortable in your clothes? Will it give you more energy? Will you sleep better? Will you laugh more? Will you be happier? Will you be a better wife or mum? Attempt to get as thorough and realistic as possible. How will your life change if you change your lifestyle?

Take time to visualize a better life initially and throughout your weight loss plan. Changing your habits is hard, so why bother if it doesn't bring you something new and better? Imagine a better life that will give you something to look forward to and work towards. See what you want, and get a picture of it. Vision is going to direct your life.

The "Law of Thinking" of Bob Proctor states: "The Law of Thinking dictates that we can only attract what we think. By changing your conscious thought pattern, which is your ruling state, you will allow yourself to change the result to what you want effectively. How far a person can go or how great the success a person can have depends on the thinking." "Visualization is where everything starts."

Believe You Are in Control

You must realize you control your life. You must take responsibility for your actions to excel in losing weight and other goals; you must trust that you are in charge. You can never move on if you put your future in other people's hands. Of course, circumstances are always out of our control, but your reaction is up to you.

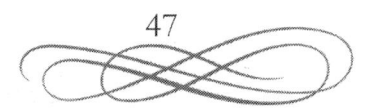

While taking control of your life is empowering, it's also frightening because if you don't achieve your goal, you have no one to blame but yourself. "No one has control over your life but you."

Get to Learn How to Cope

Many of your problems with weight loss are from your physiological reactions to stress. Most times, you crave spaghetti or candy when you have a bad day. Or you order a pizza because there is nothing to cook for dinner. Or you give up on losing weight when work gets busy or when you get to some other stressful season of life.

When you want to lose weight, life doesn't just continue effortlessly without stress. Sadly, life will never be secure, and pain will always exist. Consequently, if you fall off track each time life does not go your way, then it is time you learn new coping strategies. The goal is to maintain a healthy lifestyle and lose weight, no matter the obstacles life throws us.

If how you cope with stress keeps you from putting new behaviors in place or maintaining them, you might want to talk to a therapist or counselor. A therapist or psychologist will help you develop healthier coping skills and work through stress. It will help you free up space in your brain to focus on that better life. Having excellent optimistic coping skills is necessary for growth and survival, not just weight loss. Life is unpredictable and will not always go according to plan. Either you can get better or get bitter.

"The secret of success is learning to use pain and pleasure instead of having pain and pleasure use you. If you do that, you're in control of your life. If you don't, life controls you." - Tony Robbins.

Eliminate the Clutter and the Chaos

What do clutter and chaos have to do with weight loss? It's tough to picture a happier future surrounded by confusion and noise. Clutter and confusion build hot zones, and developing new patterns and behaviors is challenging when attempting to escape them. Hot zones are when you feel stressed and overwhelmed, and your decisions are more about surviving the moment than long-term goals.

Concentrate on Solutions and Not Explanations

A proactive approach that has been effective in weight loss is relying on options instead of excuses. You may be using excuses because you're scared of failing. So, you say something like, "I can't get to the gym at that time," or "I'm sick," or "That exercise never worked for me," instead of falling into an exercise routine. It offers you the freedom to either give up or not try. Failure, however, is part of the process. Failure is good. And instead of making yourself give up, grant yourself the approval to lose. To succeed, you must be okay with failure, not just at losing weight but in life.

Say Thank You

It's so crucial to express gratitude for everything life offers us. Feeling thankful makes us humble and appreciative of our struggles to accomplish goals. It says thank you to the universe and recognizes all of your efforts.

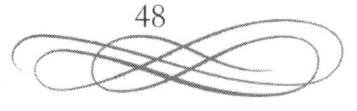

If you're trying to change habits or work past hard times, take time every day and talk about 1-3 things for which you're grateful, like genuine thanks. Talk of the lessons learned and how, because of that, you will get stronger. Life is short or long, and being thankful will help you appreciate everything you have rather than focusing on the negative. Your life will change just by thinking more positively.

"Gratitude is a powerful process for shifting your energy and bringing more of what you want into your life. Be grateful for what you already have, and you will attract more good things." - Bob Proctor.

Talk With Your Doctor

Any improvement in lifestyle should be made with the feedback from your doctor. There will be many blogs selling the perfect diet. However, the fact is that our bodies are different, and the needs of everyone are diverse. Make sure to talk to a professional with knowledge of your medical history to get the best results in your attempt to begin a healthy lifestyle. They can thus help you in making the right choices for you. Your doctor may recommend a healthy heart diet if you have high cholesterol. Or they might recommend a higher calorie intake if you are incredibly active in supporting your exercise. Regardless, you should never change your eating habits without consulting your primary care physician first.

Other Changes in Lifestyle Which Promote Healthy Eating

Here are some further tips for changing your eating patterns with that in mind:

Get Enough Sleep

An essential part of any good lifestyle is the proper amount of sleep. You cannot realize that, but having only 30 minutes less sleep than your body demands will reduce your energy and motivation to exercise. Simultaneously, too much sleep also correlates with a slower metabolism, as it reduces the number of calories you consume daily. Find a happy average and stick to it like the recommended seven to nine hours. When you are full of functional strength, you will quickly find committing to a healthy lifestyle is simpler.

Don't Over-Rely on Exercise

Ancient wisdom says the more you exercise, the more you can eat. This may not necessarily be true. Studies have shown that what you eat affects your health much more than how much you exercise. And while you want to make sure you eat enough to help your workout routine, frequent workouts don't offer your carte blanche to eat anything you want. However, that doesn't mean the workout is not essential either. A healthy, active habit that includes at least one hour of exercise each day is the best way to ensure that the improvements in your lifestyle will have the effects you are searching for.

How You Can Tell Change Is Happening

Embarking on a lifestyle change is a marathon, not a sprint. You're in it for the long haul, aiming for lasting transformation rather than instant gratification. Yet, understandably, you yearn to see the fruits of your labor. How do you gauge if your efforts are truly paying off?

Reflect on your mindset after dedicating a couple of months to this journey. Notice any shifts? And remember, indulging in a treat shouldn't stir up guilt. If you're adopting a healthy approach to eating, enjoying a scoop of ice cream as a reward for a week of nutritious meals won't make you a failure.

As your perspective evolves, so will your eating habits. You'll find yourself eating just enough to satisfy your hunger, without the urge to finish off every last crumb simply because it's there. This is a sign of true progress.

Revisit your initial journal entries and compare them to your current thoughts on health and life. It's not just about tightening your belt a notch but the overall positive impact on your wellbeing.

A life rich in wellness, good food, and relaxation isn't about looking good in swimwear; it's about fostering happiness and fulfillment over a lifetime. The key? Embrace changes that are sustainable, not just quick fixes that distract from deeper, lasting improvements. Remember, your results are a mirror of your mindset. Shift your thinking, and a healthier, happier you will follow.

This philosophy extends to your eating habits, especially with Intermittent Fasting. When your eating window opens, you'll naturally gravitate towards foods that nourish and satisfy, leaving little room for junk. Over time, your body will prefer these healthier choices, making "treats" less appealing.

But keep this in mind: transformation doesn't happen overnight. It's a gradual process of reshaping your habits and mindset. So, be patient with yourself and allow time for these changes to take root.

Best Home Exercise During Your IF

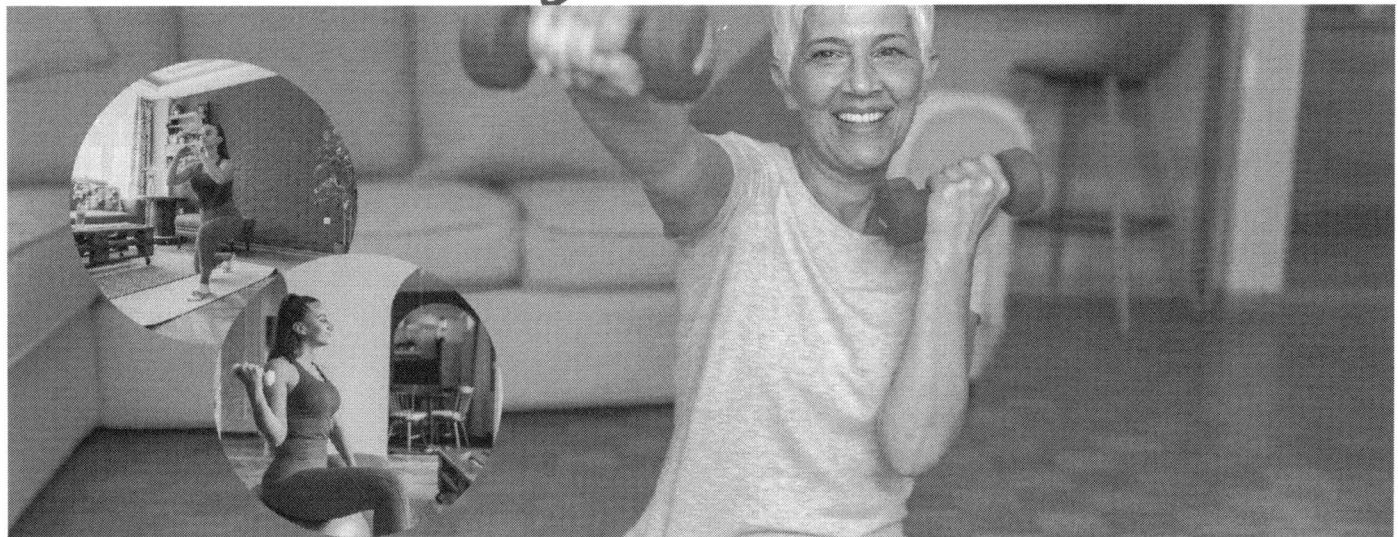

Integrating exercise into your intermittent fasting regimen can significantly enhance its benefits, from boosting metabolism to improving insulin sensitivity. Having that said, here are some exercises to give your intermittent fast a major boost. You can find the video execution of these exercises on the website dedicated to this book. You can find the link on page 102.

Weightlifting

- **Core Benefits**: Helps in maintaining and even increasing muscle mass during fasting periods, crucial for preventing muscle loss as we age.
- **Fasting and Fat Loss**: Acts as a double-edged sword by preserving muscle while primarily burning fat for energy, making it a critical component for those aiming for weight loss or body composition improvements.
- **Practical Tips**: Focus on compound movements like squats, deadlifts, and bench presses for maximum efficiency. Begin with lighter weights to assess energy levels and gradually increase intensity.

Pushups

- **Metabolic Enhancer**: A staple bodyweight exercise that effectively increases heart rate and engages multiple muscle groups simultaneously, leading to higher metabolic rates.
- **Fasting Friendly**: Performing a moderate number of pushups can significantly impact

fat metabolism without overtaxing the body's energy reserves during fasting.

- **Variations for Effectiveness**: Incorporate different pushup variations (e.g., wide, narrow, incline) to target muscles differently and prevent plateauing.

Running/Treadmill

- **Cardiovascular Boost**: Running, especially in the early fasting hours, enhances cardiovascular efficiency and accelerates fat burning by tapping into fat stores for energy.
- **Optimal Timing**: Engage in running during the first third of the fasting window to leverage the body's residual energy stores, ensuring a balance between energy expenditure and fasting benefits.
- **Mindful Running**: Listen to your body's signals, keeping hydration in focus, and adjust pace and distance based on how you feel on any given day.

Squats

- **Lower Body and Core Strengthener**: Targets the glutes, quads, hamstrings, and core, promoting fat loss in the lower body and improving overall strength and stability.
- **Technique Matters**: Maintain correct form by keeping feet shoulder-width apart, back straight, and lowering into a squat position as if sitting back into a chair, ensuring knees don't extend past toes.
- **Progression and Variation**: Add weights or try different squat variations (e.g., sumo, goblet, split) to increase intensity and target different muscle groups.

Dips

- **Upper Body Intensifier**: Excellent for targeting the triceps, shoulders, and chest, dips enhance upper body strength and contribute to a more defined muscle tone.
- **Execution**: Use parallel bars or a stable surface, keeping elbows tucked and descending until arms are at least at a 90-degree angle before pushing back up.
- **Adaptation**: Beginners can start with bench dips, gradually progressing to parallel bar dips as strength increases.

Reverse Lunge

- **Balance and Coordination**: Improves lower body strength, focusing on the glutes and hamstrings, while enhancing balance and muscular coordination.
- **Form and Function**: Step back into a lunge, maintaining a straight back and lowering the hips until the front thigh is parallel to the floor, ensuring the knee doesn't overshoot the toes.
- **Variability for Growth**: Introduce weights or switch to walking lunges for added challenge and to prevent adaptation.

Planks

- **Core Stability Powerhouse**: Strengthens the entire core, supporting spinal health and improving posture, with extensive benefits for overall movement efficiency.

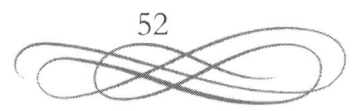

- **Consistency is Key**: Maintain a straight line from head to heels, engaging the core to prevent hips from sagging or piking up.
- **Variations for Challenge**: Experiment with side planks, forearm planks, or add movement (e.g., plank jacks, shoulder taps) to increase difficulty and engage different muscle groups.

Burpee

- **All-in-One Workout**: Combines a squat, pushup, and jump into one fluid movement, offering a high-intensity, full-body workout that spikes the metabolism.
- **Strategic Integration**: Perfect for HIIT sessions during fasting to maximize fat burn and cardiovascular benefits, but monitor energy levels to avoid overexertion.
- **Modifications for All Levels**: Adjust the intensity by removing the jump or pushup for a less strenuous version, gradually building up to the full movement.

Yoga

- **Holistic Approach**: Balances physical fitness with mental well-being, offering hormonal balance, stress reduction, and flexibility improvements, making it an ideal complement to fasting.
- **Diverse Styles**: From gentle Hatha to more intense Vinyasa or Ashtanga, there's a yoga style to match every fitness level and goal.
- **Accessibility**: With minimal equipment needed, yoga can be practiced anywhere, emphasizing the importance of breath control and mindfulness.
- **Benefits**: Enhances organ oxygenation and detoxifies, improves posture and flexibility, tones muscles, boosts circulation, and regulates breathing. It also lowers blood pressure, stabilizes blood sugar, increases bone density, aids digestion, and activates the parasympathetic nervous system.

Walking the Stairs

- **Efficiency**: Allows you to improve the health of your heart and lungs, has a low impact on the joints, and is useful for developing speed, power, and agility.
- **Convenience**: No special equipment needed, can be performed in various settings.

General Tips

Exercising while fasting can boost your metabolic rate, enhance insulin sensitivity, and aid in fat loss. It's important to select physical activities that align with your energy levels and personal preferences to ensure consistency and maximize the benefits of combining fasting with exercise.

Best Apps for Your IF

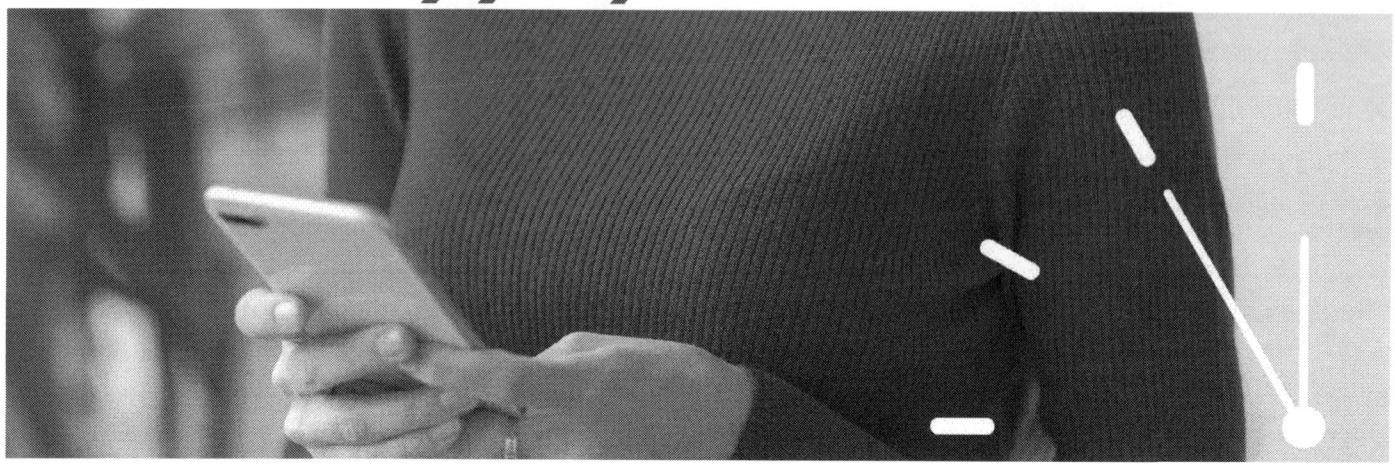

In this chapter, I want to introduce some apps to help you during your Intermittent Fasting. Each app has its particularity, and it's worth trying at least a couple to see which fits best for your needs. I preferred not to list pricing information for the various subscription plans here, as they could change quite often and could have been misleading.

You'll find links to download the apps, with other up-to-date information, on the website dedicated to this book. You can find the link on page 1026.

Ate Food Journal

Ate Food Diary is useful for keeping a visually striking food diary. It shows how much time has passed between meals to increase awareness about what you ate and how it made you feel. If you're into social media, you can easily share what you've eaten with Ate Food Diary.

The free version of the app lasts only 7 days, and a monthly or yearly subscription is required to continue using the app.

BodyFast

BodyFast lets you choose from as many as 10 different IF plans. It offers some interesting tips, even from a dietary perspective. BodyFast makes suggestions based on your age and weight (current and loss goals), but you have to be careful what it suggests since it's software, not a doctor.

There's a free version and a paid version of this app.

DoFasting

DoFasting allows you to choose from seven IF plans. It also offers many informative articles, workout videos, and over 5,000 recipes.

You can create a daily, weekly, or monthly food plan to compare it to your recommended calorie intake.

It's free in the basic version. It has various subscription options: monthly, quarterly, or semi-annual.

FastHabit

Are you constantly changing your IF plan? If so, FastHabit is right for you. You can set the fasting window you want and have it start counting.
You can set reminders, statistics, and more.
This app there is also a free version and a paid one

Fastic

Fastic contains many recipes with healthy, filling foods to make the most of the intervals you can eat. It tells you what is happening to your body while fasting and has a fasting timer and step counter inside. There's also a community of "fasting buddies," which can help find the right motivation.
This app is also available in both free and paid versions.

Fastient

If you want to keep track of your fasting times, Fastient is among the most comprehensive apps. You can record what you eat and see the progress you're making. The clear interface shows simple graphs that help you monitor your progress.
There is a free version and also an annual or lifetime subscription.

LIFE Intermittent Fast Tracker

Whatever your IF plan is, LIFE Intermittent Fast Tracker will work for you. It allows you to set up fasting windows in a completely customized way. If you're also doing the ketogenic diet, this app helps track how long you've been in ketosis. Additionally, you can connect with other app users to fast and motivate each other.
Again, there's a free and a paid version.

Simple

As you can guess from the name, Simple is a minimalist app. The IF plan is fully customizable, and the app offers expert tips to help you with your IF. It can connect to your iPhone's Health app to track your weight, steps, etc.
The basic version is free, and a paid version with monthly, quarterly, or yearly subscriptions.

Vora

Vora's strong point is community support. It can be a very important, almost indispensable support for someone. Especially for long-term goals, having a community with which to confront is very useful in not losing motivation.
Vora is available with a free and paid plan.

Window

Window has many features to simplify your Intermittent Fasting. You can schedule the intervals in which you can eat, and you'll be notified when the eating interval has started or when it's about to end (very convenient for having one last snack). Inside there is a blog with various tips on wellness and nutrition. It's certainly the best solution for those who have just started.
The basic app is free, and a premium version is available.

Zero

Zero allows you to customize this app by tracking your fasting times. It alerts you when it's time to eat! It's a simple and minimalist app that helps you analyze your eating habits over time. It can connect with your FitBit or Oura ring.
The app is free; you can do a monthly or yearly subscription.

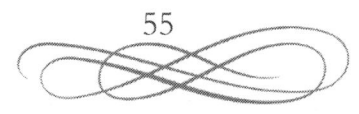

FAQ

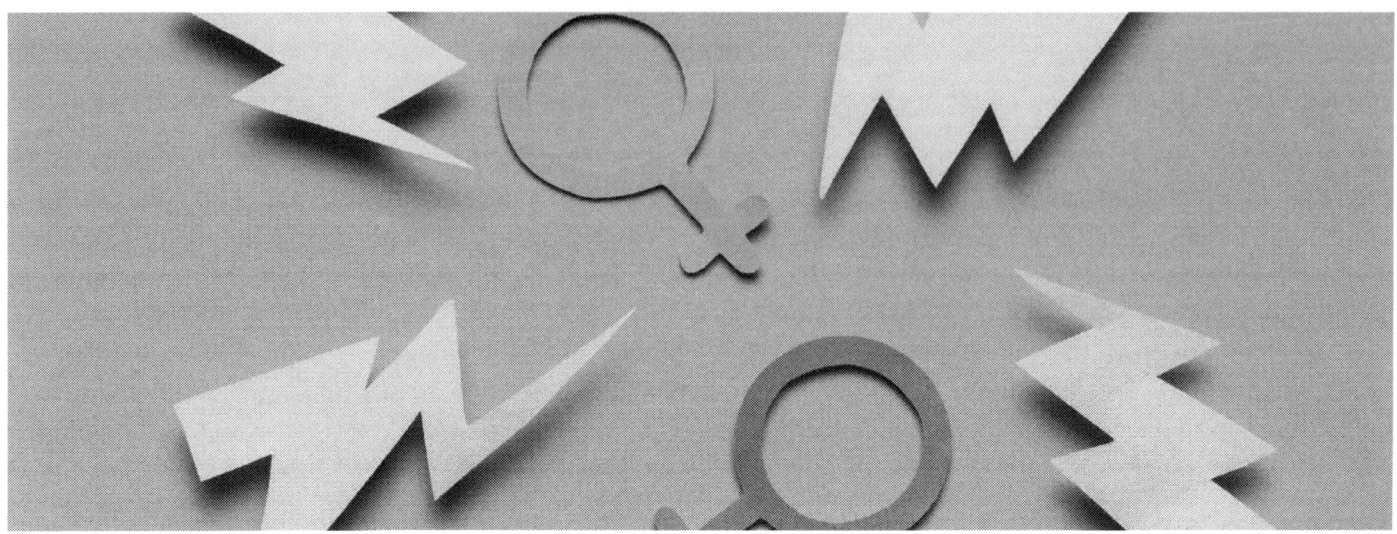

Fasting can be difficult at times, and we know it! There are certain concerns that every beginner gets after opting for Intermittent Fasting. The following frequently asked questions can help resolve basic queries about fasting and its effects on health.

#1: What Can I Eat or Drink During Fasting?

As we said earlier, to reap the full benefits of Intermittent Fasting, you shouldn't eat or drink anything with calories.

On the other hand, we also argue that small amounts of good fats will not hinder your goals if you only want to control your insulin.

And finally, we also say that some authors defend the idea that eating very few calories (up to 50 kcal) would not break your fast, regardless of the source of those calories.

Even so, some people prefer a summary list of foods to help them get started.

This practical list helps to remember which foods and drinks can or cannot be consumed during the prompt window without necessarily "breaking your fast" or ending all its benefits.

For this reason, we have compiled a short, non-exhaustive list of foods that can be eaten without disturbing your fast.

#2: What About Sweetened Foods but No Calories? Like Coffee with Stevia, Erythritol or Sucralose, and Even Zero Soda?

By now, you have understood that Intermittent Fasting is not consuming food so as not to ingest calories or raise insulin.

So, using non-caloric sweeteners should be allowed, right?

Calm down. This issue is more complex than it may seem at first.

First, I strongly recommend you understand the differences between low-carb sweeteners.

But, as we explained, we still have an important question, even if we consider only sweeteners that do not raise insulin (as is the case with stevia, or even erythritol, for example).

Although this relationship is speculative — unproven— there are possibly several potential mechanisms through which sweeteners can interfere with metabolism.

And that even includes interactions with sweet taste receptors, which would stimulate other metabolic adaptations.

Certainly, more research is needed, but this is yet another sign that it can be smart not to abuse sweeteners.

In our opinion, one thing is certain: the daily consumption of sweeteners is not ideal for your health, even though it may not hinder weight loss or break your fast.

This situation is valid in the case of artificial sweeteners and even more so in the case of zero-calorie soft drinks.

#3: Who Can Do Intermittent Fasting?

When discussing fasting and its benefits, people often have an important question: precisely who can and cannot fast (practice it).

The direct answer is that Intermittent Fasting is suitable for healthy adults.

It is even easier to discuss who should not start fasting without first talking to their trusted doctor.

#4: Does Fasting Slow Metabolism?

If you are paying attention to this text, you should already intuitively know the answer.

No, Intermittent Fasting does not slow down metabolism.

The keyword in this sentence is "intermittent."

Spending long periods (several days) without eating will imply a metabolic adaptation (that is, a slowing down of the metabolism).

A very long and/or severe caloric restriction will also have the same effect.

It happens because our body seeks to survive above all else.

So, if you go without eating for several days, your body will seek to preserve energy.

However, on short fasts, our metabolism tends to increase.

In this case, one study found a 3.6% increase in metabolism on short fasts, and another found that metabolism increased by 10% during fasting.

It makes evolutionary sense: if our body seeks to feed, it needs to stimulate us and not deprive us of our energy —so that we can hunt/collect food and thus obtain energy.

It is probably mediated by hormonal changes during fasting, such as increased adrenaline.

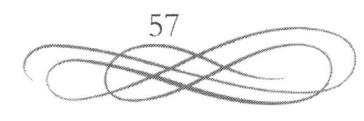

#5: Intermittent Fasting Causes Loss of Muscle Mass (Lean Mass)?

Another very common question is regarding the conservation of muscle mass when we practice fasting.

This question arises mainly because we always hear around (especially repeated as a mantra in gyms) that if you don't eat every three hours, your body will start to burn muscles to provide you with energy.

Unfortunately, this myth is very common, and we have no idea where it originated.

If you read the question about "eating every 3 hours" we answered above, you will understand that you don't have to eat every 3 hours to conserve your muscle mass.

On the other hand, you may wonder if taking longer periods without eating (16, 24, 48 hours, or more) would damage your lean mass.

But you can rest easy: during the fasting window, you will not break muscles as a form of energy.

Your muscles can even serve as an energy source, but you have other reserves that are much easier for your body to use, such as fat in your belly and elsewhere and glycogen.

Remember that glycogen is our energy reserve in the form of carbohydrates, stored both in the liver and muscles, between the muscle cells.

#6: Can I Exercise During Fasting?

Another very common question concerns fasting and physical exercise.

The most common questions are:

1. Can I train while fasting?
2. Can I not eat anything after training?
3. Can I train while fasting and continue to fast afterward?

The answer to these questions and their variations is: you can do whatever you want.

You can train on a fast if you feel good, for example.

At the same time, some people may not feel well; in this case, they shouldn't be training fasting.

Of course, if you're on a high-carb, especially refined diet, eating every three hours for a low-carb diet and still starting fasting and training hard, it's normal that you will not feel well.

You need to give your body time to adapt to all these changes.

However, we believe that most people can train while fasting after some adaptation if they want to.

That is, there is nothing special about fasting that prevents you from training.

You can even practice fasting and fast for a few more hours until your lunch.

As we mentioned, in the case of lean gains fasting, you don't necessarily need to have your first meal right before or right after your workout.

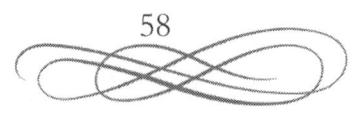

#7: Which Supplements Do Not Break Intermittent Fasting?

Now that you know you can train on an empty stomach without eating anything before and nothing afterward, maybe your next question is precisely related to supplements.

As we have said before, theoretically, fasting is when you should not eat anything.

However, there are exceptions, as in the case of insulin fasting.

So, it is natural that doubts related to supplements arise as well, especially because there are supplements that do not break fast because they do not contain calories.

#8: Can I Take Bone Broth?

First, what is bone broth, and why would anyone want it?

In short, bone broth is the drink obtained by boiling the bones and connective tissue of different types of animals.

It is rich in vitamins, minerals, collagen, and other nutrients.

And it happens because the bone broth is rich in nutrients; it becomes interesting for longer fasts. It can replace nutrients (vitamins and minerals) lost during the fasting window.

After all, you frequently eliminate water and minerals during this period through urine and sweat.

#9: What to Say When Someone Criticizes Your Fasting?

The truth is that, even with all the support that science gives to this practice, fasting is still a controversial topic for most people. As strange as it may be, we live in a society where skipping meals occasionally and eating real food is considered controversial.

So, don't be alarmed if you receive unwanted criticism or comments from friends and family.

Breakfast Recipes

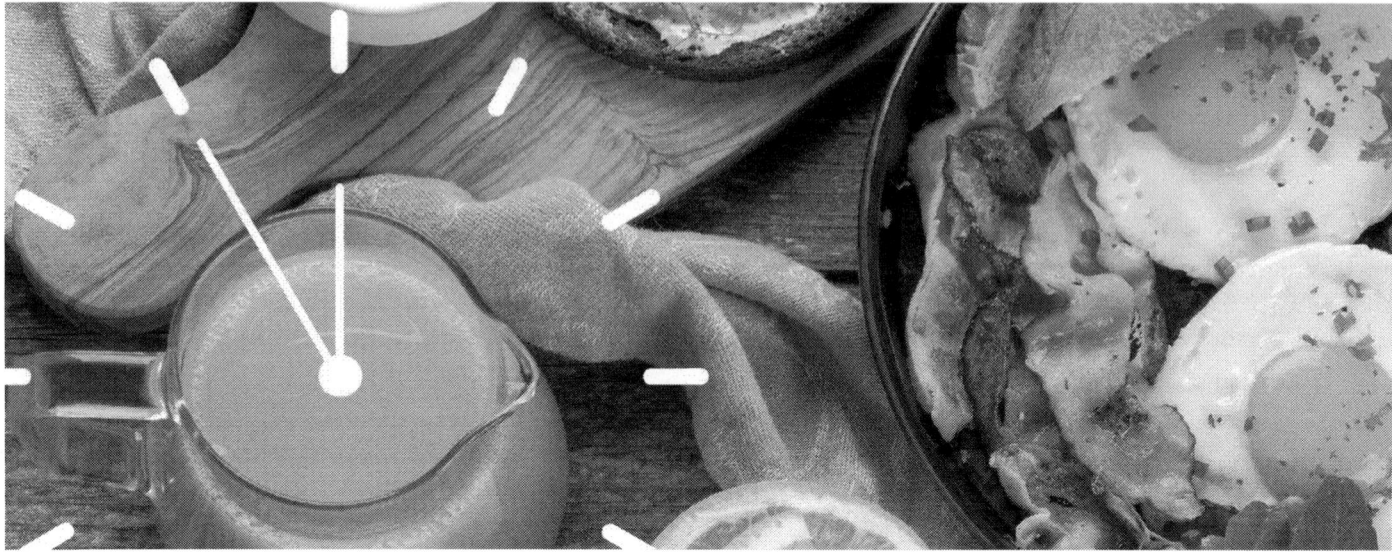

Refer to the end of the book for the conversion chart.

40-Second Omelet
Time: 25 Mins, Serves: 1, Skill: Easy

Ingredients
- Eggs (2)
- Water (2 tbsp)
- Filling (vegetables, meat, seafood) (1/2 cup)
- Unsalted butter (1 tbsp)

Instructions
- Combine the eggs and water in a mixing bowl and whisk until smooth.
- Melt the butter in a 10" omelet pan/frypan until a water drop sizzles.
- Pour the egg mixture into the pan, quickly spreading it out on the sides, and using an inverted pancake turner, carefully push cooked portions from the edges to the center, allowing uncooked portions to come into contact with the heated pan's surface. Tilt and move the pan as desired.
- If necessary, fill the omelet with 1/2 cup beef, vegetables, or seafood filling, placing the filling on the left side if you're right-handed and on the right side if you're left-handed.
- Invert the bottom half of the omelet onto a plate using the pancake turner.

Mexican Egg & Veggie Skillet
Time: 25 Mins, Serves: 4, Skill: Easy

Ingredients
- Eggs (8)
- Zucchini or bell peppers, thinly sliced (1 cup)
- Butter (2 tbsp)
- Low salt sugar-free ketchup (1/4 cup)
- Chili powder (1 tsp)
- Green onions (2), sliced thin

Instructions
- Whisk the eggs together in a mixing bowl until well combined.
- Mix ketchup, chili powder, and green onions with the egg mixture.
- In a pan, melt the butter, then add the thinly sliced zucchini or bell peppers and cook over medium heat until slightly tender.

- Pour in the egg mixture, scramble until you reach the desired consistency.
- Serve right away on warm plates.

Stuffed Breakfast Veggie Cups
Time: 40 Mins, Serves: 4, Skill: Easy

Ingredients
- Eggs (4)
- Reduced-sodium bacon (8 oz.), cooked and crumbled
- Cheddar cheese (1 cup), shredded
- Scallions (1/4 cup), thinly sliced

Instructions
- Preheat the oven to 375°F.
- Whisk the eggs in a bowl.
- Grease a muffin tin and pour the whisked eggs into each cup until halfway full.
- Add bacon, cheese, and scallions to each cup.
- Bake for 15-20 minutes or until the eggs are set

Cheesesteak Quiche
Time: 50 Mins, Serves: 6, Skill: Easy

Ingredients
- Eggs, beaten (5)
- Cream (1 cup)
- Prepared Almond flour crust (1" x 9")
- Black pepper (1/2 tsp)
- Coarsely chopped Sirloin steak meat (1/2 lb.)
- Onions (1 cup), diced
- Canola oil (2 tbsp)
- Shredded pepper jack cheese (1/2 cup)

Instructions
- Cut the sliced sirloin into coarse pieces.
- Brown the sliced steak and onions in a sauté pan with the oil, then set aside to cool for 10 minutes before folding in the cheese and letting it rest.
- Whisk the eggs, cream, and black pepper in a large mixing cup until thoroughly combined.
- Spread the steak and cheese mixture on the bottom of the par-cooked almond flour crust, then top with the egg mixture and bake at 350°F for 30 minutes.
- Cover the cheesesteak quiche with foil and turn off the oven for 10 minutes before serving.

Homemade Low-Carb Muesli
Time: 55 Mins, Serves: 5, Skill: Medium

Ingredients
- Chopped nuts (almonds, pecans, macadamia) (1 cup)
- Fresh berries (1/2 cup)
- Chia seeds (1/4 cup)
- Stevia or monk fruit sweetener (to taste)

Instructions
- In a mixing bowl, combine chopped nuts, chia seeds, and fresh berries.
- Sweeten with stevia or monk fruit to taste.
- Serve with almond milk or non-dairy yogurt.

Low-Carb Egg Sandwich
Time: 25 Mins, Serves: 4, Skill: Easy

Ingredients
- Egg (1)
- Water (1 tbsp)
- Cheddar cheese (1 slice)
- Large lettuce leaves or homemade cloud bread (2 pieces)
- Basil leaves (3 meds)
- Olive oil (1/2 tbsp)
- Tomato (2 slices)

Instructions
- Heat olive oil in a small skillet over medium heat.
- Whisk the egg with water, season with salt and pepper.
- Cook the egg in the skillet, forming an omelet.
- Assemble the sandwich with lettuce leaves or cloud bread, cheese, cooked egg, tomato slices, and basil leaves..

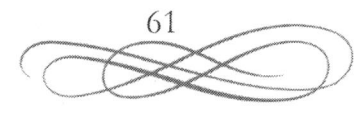

Southern Style Cauliflower Grits
Time: 55 Mins, Serves: 2, Skill: Medium

Ingredients
- Cauliflower, riced (2 cups)
- Milk (1/3 cup) - choose almond or coconut milk for lower carbs
- Butter (1 tbsp)
- Salt and pepper to taste
- Cheddar cheese, shredded (optional)

Instructions
- In a saucepan, combine riced cauliflower, milk, and half the butter.
- Cook over medium heat for 10-15 minutes, stirring frequently until cauliflower is soft.
- Stir in remaining butter, season with salt and pepper.
- Add cheese if desired, stirring until melted.

Almond & Berry Overnight "No-Oats"
Time: 25 Mins, Serves: 1, Skill: Easy

Ingredients
- Almond milk (1/2 cup)
- Stevia or monk fruit sweetener (to taste)
- Cinnamon (1/8 tsp)
- Chia seeds (1/4 cup)
- Almond flour (1/4 cup)
- Berries of your choice (1/2 cup)

Instructions
- In a mason jar, mix almond milk, chia seeds, almond flour, and cinnamon.
- Sweeten with stevia or monk fruit.
- Add berries, stir well to combine.
- Refrigerate overnight.

Spicy Almond Mix
Time: 30 Mins, Serves: 2, Skill: Easy

Ingredients
- Almonds and pecans (4 cups)
- Olive oil (1/2 cup)
- Chili powder (1 tbsp)
- Cayenne pepper (dash)
- Ground cumin (1/2 tsp)

Instructions
- Preheat oven to 300°F.
- Toss nuts with olive oil and spices until evenly coated.
- Spread on a baking sheet and roast for 15-20 minutes, stirring occasionally..

Low-Carb Burritos with Eggs and Mexican Sausage
Time: 25 Mins, Serves: 4, Skill: Easy

Ingredients
- Eggs, beaten (3)
- Low-carb tortillas or large lettuce leaves (3)
- Chorizo (3 oz.)

Instructions
- In a skillet, cook the chorizo until browned.
- Stir in the eggs, scramble until cooked through.
- Place the egg

Vegetable Recipes

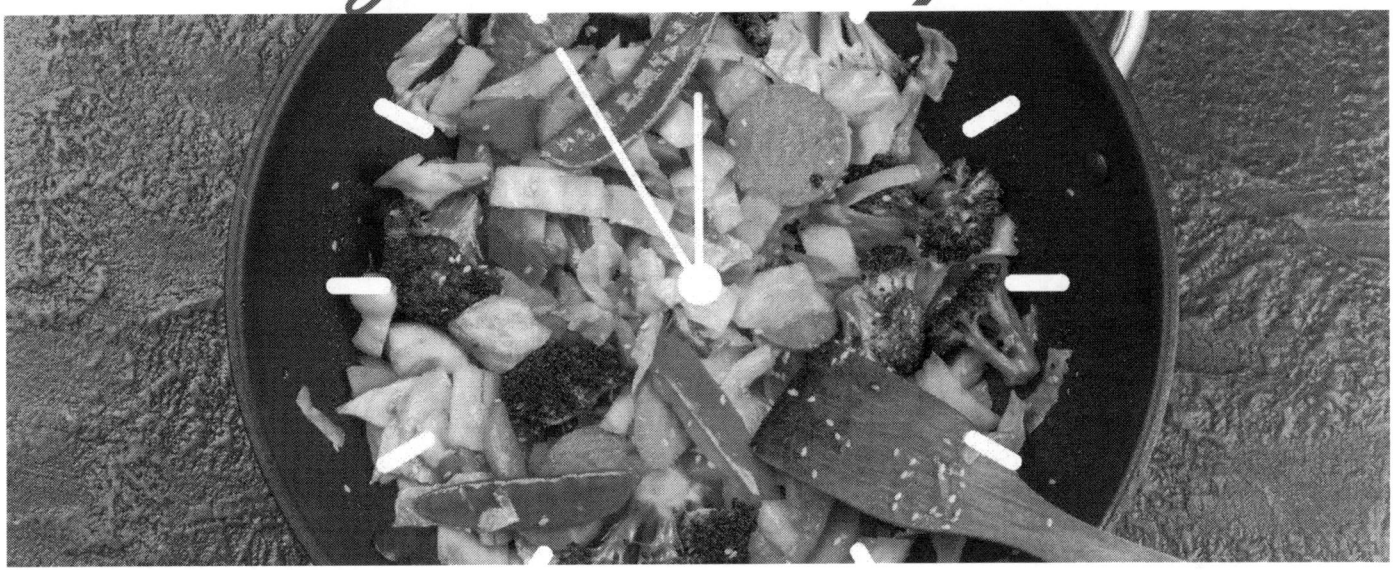

Refer to the end of the book for the conversion chart.

Italian Eggplant Salad
Time: 25 Mins, Serves: 4, Skill: Easy

Ingredients
- Black pepper (1/4 tsp)
- Tomato (1 med), chopped
- Olive oil (3 tbsp)
- Eggplant (3 cups), cubed
- Onion (1 small), chopped
- White wine vinegar (2 tbsp)
- Garlic clove (1), chopped
- Oregano (1/2 tsp)

Instructions
- Put the eggplant in a pot of water that has been brought to a simmer.
- Bring the water to a boil and then reduce the heat.
- Cook for a further 10 minutes with the saucepan lid on.
- Drain the eggplants and place them in serving dishes with the onions and tomato.
- In a shallow dish, combine the garlic, oregano, vinegar, and black pepper.
- Combine the onions, tomato, and eggplant with the vinegar mixture.
- Drizzle a little oil over the eggplant mixture before serving.

Mix Berry Coleslaw
Time: 1 hour 15 Mins, Serves: 3, Skill: Easy

Ingredients
- Mix berries (raspberries, blackberries) (2 cups) washed and drained
- Cabbage (2 cups), shredded
- Greek yogurt (1/4 cup)
- Pepper, to taste
- Onion (1/4 cup), chopped

Instructions
- In a large mixing cup, combine the cabbage, yogurt, mix berries, pepper, and onion.
- Chill for 60 minutes before serving.

Roasted tomatillo salsa
Time: 45 Mins, Serves: 8, Skill: Medium

Ingredients
- Lime juice (1/4 cup)
- Cilantro (1 bunch)
- Water (1/4 cup)
- Tomatillos (17)
- Head garlic (1)
- Jalapenos (3)

Instructions
- Start by slicing the tomatillos.
- In a greased baking pan, mix the tomatillos, jalapenos, and garlic.
- To simmer in water, put them in the oven for 15 minutes.
- In a processor, puree the cooked tomatillo mixture with lime juice and cilantro until creamy.

Smoothie bowl
Time: 20 Mins, Serves: 1, Skill: Easy

Ingredients
- Blackberries (1 tbsp), fresh
- Unsweetened coconut (1 tbsp), shredded
- Protein powder (2 tbsp)
- Avocado (1/2)
- Raspberries (1 cup), frozen
- Water (1/4 cup)
- Coconut milk (3 tbsp)
- Stevia (1 tsp)

Instructions
- In a high-powered blender, combine the avocado, water, raspberries, coconut milk, protein powder, and stevia to make a smooth sorbet.
- Put the sorbet into a cup and top with fresh blackberries and coconut before ready to consume.
- After pouring the mixture into the serving dish, serve with tacos.

Vegan shortbread cookies
Time: 55 Mins, Serves: 8, Skill: Medium

Ingredients
- Coconut oil (1/4 cup)
- Mixed nuts (almonds, cashew, pecans) (1/4 cup), chopped
- Baking soda (1/8 tsp)
- Coconut flour (1 cup)
- Sunflower seeds (1/8 cup), grinded
- Stevia (1/2 cup)
- Non-dairy yogurt (2 1/2 tbsp)
- Vanilla extract (1 tsp)
- Cardamom (1 tsp), ground
- Almond flour (1/2 cup)
- Salt (1/4 teaspoon)

Instructions
- Preheat the oven to 325 °F.
- Whisk together yogurt, stevia, and coconut oil, then include cardamom and vanilla to produce a creamy and smooth mixture.
- In a mixing cup, add the flour, salt, and baking soda.
- In a mixing bowl, combine the flour mix and coconut oil mix. To produce a dough, mix the ingredients together with a spoon.
- Combine the nuts and seeds in the dough. Thoroughly knead the dough.
- Make a log out of the dough.
- After covering the logs with parchment paper, place them in the freezer for 30 minutes.
- Cut the logs after they've been frozen and put them in a baking tray lined with parchment paper.
- Bake the cake for 20 minutes, or until baked through.
- Keep in an airtight container after baking.

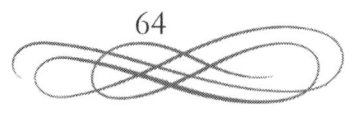

Crepes with blueberries
Time: 1 hour and 5 Mins, Serves: 4, Skill: Hard

Ingredients
For crepes:
- Butter (1 1/2 tbsp)
- Flaxseed flour (1 cup)
- Coconut milk (1 1/4 cups)
- Large eggs (2)

For sauce:
- Stevia (1/2 cup)
- Blueberry pulp (3/4 cup)

Instructions
- In a mixing bowl, whisk together the eggs, milk, and flour. Set the bowl aside.
- In a saucepan, combine the stevia and berry pulp.
- Over medium heat, bring the berry pulp mixture to a simmer.
- Reduce the heat to low and continue to cook until the liquid has been reduced to half its original volume. Set it aside for the time being.
- In a crepe tray, melt half a tablespoon of butter over high heat, then pour in crepe batter and spread it out. Cook for about 1 ½ minutes on one side. Cook for another 45 seconds after flipping the crepe.
- When the crepe is finished, transfer it to a serving plate and top it with a spoonful of sauce before folding it in half and serving.

Festive Cranberry Stuffing
Time: 45 Mins, Serves: 2, Skill: Easy

Ingredients
- Sugar-free cranberry juice (1/4 cup)
- Stale coconut flour bread (3 cups)
- Poultry seasoning (1/4 tsp)
- Raw cranberries (1/2 cup)
- Rhubarb stalks (1 cup), finely chopped
- Celery (1/4 cup), chopped
- Unsalted butter (2 tablespoons)

Instructions
- Combine stale coconut flour bread, rhubarb stalks, sugar-free cranberry juice, celery, cranberries, poultry seasoning, and butter in a large mixing bowl.
- Bake for 30 minutes at 350 °F in a preheated oven after pouring the batter into a greased casserole dish.

Simple Puerto Rican sofrito
Time: 35 Mins, Serves: 2, Skill: Easy

Ingredients
- Culantro (6 leaves), opt
- Cilantro (1 bunch)
- Garlic cloves (10), chopped
- Green pepper (1), chopped
- Salt (1 tsp)
- Aja peppers (5)
- Spanish Onion (1), chopped

Instructions
- To start, in a blender, puree the onions.
- Combine the green bell pepper, garlic, culantro, dulce pepper, cilantro, and salt in the blender with the onions.
- In an airtight jar, freeze the sofrito.
- Add two teaspoons of sofrito when you are making rice, peas, or soups.

Broccoli blossom
Time: 25 Mins, Serves: 2, Skill: Easy

Ingredients
- Tarragon (1/4 tsp)
- Onion powder (1/4 tsp)
- Ground black pepper, to taste
- Oil (1 tbsp)
- Toasted English muffin or almond flour muffin (1)
- Onion (1/4 cup), chopped
- Water (3 tbsp)
- Ground red pepper, to taste
- Red cabbage (1 cup), chopped
- Garlic powder (1/4 tsp)

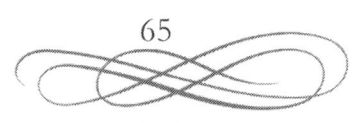

- Broccoli (1/2 cup), chopped
- Parmesan cheese (2 tbsp), grated

Instructions

- In a skillet over medium heat, heat the oil, then add the vegetables and cook for 3 minutes.
- Half-fill the skillet with water and position it over a burner to steam for 5 minutes.
- After 5 minutes, apply the spices and simmer for another 2 minutes.
- Place the vegetables on top of the muffins, serve with parmesan cheese.

Coconut curry cauliflower

Time: 37 Mins, Serves: 4, Skill: Easy

Ingredients

- Olive oil (2 tbsp)
- Lime juice (1/2 lime)
- Cauliflower (1/2 medium)
- Coconut milk (13 1/2 oz.)
- Kosher salt (1/4 tsp)
- Cilantro (1/4 cup), chopped
- Curry paste (1 tsp)

Instructions

- In a pan, heat the oil and add the salt and cauliflower. The cooking time is 7 minutes.
- Pour the coconut milk and curry paste over the cauliflower and cover the pan.
- Set the timer for 10 minutes to boil.
- Season with salt and pepper to taste and garnish with lime juice and cilantro.

Poultry Recipes

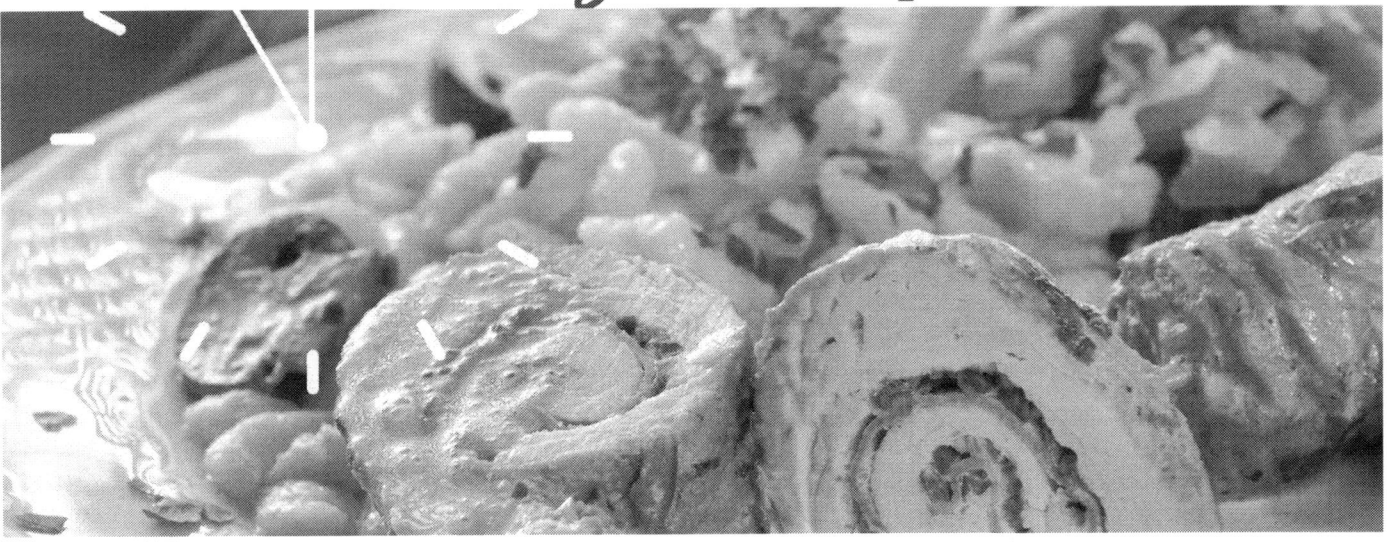

Refer to the end of the book for the conversion chart.

Chicken Veronique
Time: 40 Mins, Serves: 4, Skill: Easy

Ingredients
- Pepper (1/4 tsp)
- Water (1/2 cup)
- Orange preserves (sugar-free) (2 tbsp)
- Bay leaf (1)
- Coconut Flour (1 tbsp)
- Blueberries/Strawberries (1 cup)
- Pepper (1/4 tsp)
- Unsalted Margarine (6 tbsp)
- White wine (1/4 cup)
- Parsley (1 tsp)
- 1 chicken breast (4oz.)

Instructions
- In a mixing cup, whisk together the flour and 1/4 teaspoon of pepper. Using a thin dusting of flour, gently cover the chicken. In a pan, sauté the chicken in margarine until golden brown.
- Place the remaining components, except for the berries, in the skillet. Bring to a simmer then add the chicken. Cook for 25 minutes, or until the chicken is cooked through.
- Remove the chicken from the skillet and set aside. Cook the remaining components for a further 2 minutes, stirring continuously, while adding the berries.
- To serve, drizzle the sauce on top of the chicken.

Cauliflower-Rice Pilaf
Time: 1 Hour and 25 Mins, Serves: 3, Skill: Medium

Ingredients
- Yellow onion (1 small), chopped
- Pepper (1/8 tsp)
- Margarine (1 tbsp)
- Chicken broth (2 cups), low in sodium
- Carrot (1), peeled & chopped fine
- Stalk celery (1), chopped fine
- Cauliflower rice (1/3 cup)
- Dried thyme (1/2 tsp)

Instructions

- In a saucepan over low heat, melt the margarine, then add the onion and cook until soft, around 5 minutes.
- Add the Cauliflower rice and bring to a boil for 1 minute.
- Add the remaining ingredients and reduce to a low heat.
- Decrease the heat to low and simmer for 15 minutes, sealed, or until the liquid is gone.

Chicken Salad

Time: 1 Hour and 20 Mins, Serves: 4, Skill: Medium

Ingredients

- Chicken breasts (4), boneless & skinless
- Mayonnaise of Duke (3/4 cup)
- Raspberries (1 cup), cut in half
- Celery (1/4 cup), chopped
- Red onion (1/4 cup), chopped finely
- Salt (1/4 tsp)
- Black pepper (1/8 tsp)

Instructions

- Combine the chicken with some water in a pot. (Chicken must be covered with water.)
- Cook the chicken for 25 minutes over medium heat, then leave to cool.
- Chop the chicken into small pieces.
- Combine the raspberries, chicken, celery, mayonnaise, and onions in a bowl.
- Finish with a pinch of black pepper.

Turkey Salad

Time: 1 Hour and 10 Mins, Serves: 4, Skill: Easy

Ingredients

- Turkey breast (4), boneless & skinless
- Mayonnaise of Duke (3/4 cup)
- Raspberries (1 cup)
- Celery (1/4 cup), chopped
- Red onion (1/4 cup), chopped finely
- Salt (1/4 tsp)
- Black pepper (1/8 tsp)

Instructions

- Combine the turkey with some water in a pot. (Turkey must be covered with water.)
- Cook the turkey for 25 minutes in water over medium heat, then leave to cool.
- Chop the turkey into small pieces.
- Combine the raspberries, turkey, celery, mayonnaise, and onions in a big mixing bowl.
- Finish with a pinch of black pepper.

Curry Chicken

Time: 1 Hour and 5 Mins, Serves: 4, Skill: Medium

Ingredients

- Dry thyme (1/2 tsp)
- Lemon juice (1/4 cup)
- Onion (1 medium), chopped
- Curry powder (2 tsp)
- Black pepper (1/2 tsp)
- Garlic clove (1 medium), chopped (optional)
- Water (1 cup)
- Chicken (1 whole), cut in small parts, skin removed
- Vegetable or olive oil (2 tbsps.)

Instructions

- After cleaning the chicken, soak it with lemon juice.
- Mix the seasonings in a bowl and rub onto the chicken.
- Marinate the seasoned chicken overnight in the refrigerator.
- Heat the oil in a saucepan and brown the seasoned chicken.
- Add a splash of water to the marinating bowl to preserve marinade.
- Pour the remaining marinade over the browned chicken and cook on low heat until the chicken is tender, about 20 minutes.
- Quickly serve over hot cauliflower rice.

Easy Chicken and Pasta Dinner
Time: 1 Hour 35 Mins, Serves: 4, Skill: Medium

Ingredients
- Chicken breast (5 oz.), cooked
- Olive oil (1 tbsp)
- Red bell pepper (1/2 cup)
- Zucchini (1 cup)
- Zucchini spirals (2 cups), tenderized
- Low-sodium Italian dressing (3 tbsp)

Instructions
- Peel and thinly slice the zucchini and bell pepper.
- In a large skillet, heat the olive oil and cook the peppers and zucchini until soft and crispy, then move to a serving dish.
- Cut the chicken into small strips using a sharp knife.
- Heat the tenderized zucchini spirals and chicken strips separately in the microwave.
- Toss the spirals with the dressing and eat alongside the sautéed vegetables and chicken strips.

Chicken Waldorf salad
Time: 40 Mins, Serves: 4, Skill: Easy

Ingredients
- Miracle Whip (1/2 cup), sugar-free
- Chicken (8 oz), cooked & cubed
- Ginger (1/2 tbsp), ground, optional
- Cucumber (1/2 cup), chopped
- Fresh cranberries cranberries(2 tbsp)
- Celery (1/2 cup), chopped

Instructions
- Mix all ingredients together carefully.
- It's best to keep it in the fridge for a few hours to allow the flavors to meld.

Salisbury Steak
Time: 1 Hour 30 Mins, Serves: 4, Skill: Medium

Ingredients
- Onion (1 small), chopped
- Black pepper (1 tsp)
- Green pepper (1/2 cup), chopped
- Egg (1)
- Chopped steak, or lean ground beef (1 lb.)
- Vegetable oil (1 tbsp)
- Water (1/2 cup)
- Almond flour (1 tbsp)

Instructions
- Combine the meat, onion, black pepper, egg, and green pepper in a mixing bowl. Once mixed, shape into patties.
- In a pan, heat the oil, then add the patties and sear on all sides.
- After including half of the water, boil for 15 minutes. Remove the patties from the pan and set them aside.
- Combine the beef drippings, remaining water, and almond flour in a pan. Stir the gravy to thicken it as its heating.
- Pour the sauce over the patties and serve right away.

Basic Chicken Loaf
Time: 1 hour and 40 Mins, Serves: 4, Skill: Medium

Ingredients
- Lean chicken (1lb.), ground, boneless
- Green bell pepper (1/2 cup), diced
- Water (1/4 cup)
- Egg white (1)
- Lemon juice (1 tbsp)
- Almond flour (1/2 cup)
- Onion powder (1/2 tsp)
- Italian seasoning (1/2 tsp)
- Onions (1/2 cup), chopped
- Black pepper (1/4 tsp)

Instructions
- Preheat the oven to 200°F.
- Squeeze the juice of a lemon onto the poultry.
- Mix the remaining components in a dish.
- Gently fold in the meat.

- Cook the loaf in a skillet for 45 minutes.

Stir Fry Meal
Time: 40 Mins, Serves: 4, Skill: Easy

Ingredients
- Frozen stir fry vegetables (1 10-oz. package)
- Low sodium soy sauce (1/2 tbsp)
- Cauliflower Rice (2 cups), cooked
- Cooking oil (2 tbsp)
- Chicken breasts (2 medium), cut in bite-size pieces

Instructions
- Heat the oil in a 9x10' pan on high heat.
- Add the chicken.
- Add the vegetables and toss to combine.
- Mix thoroughly with the soy sauce.
- Lower the heat to medium-high and roast, uncovered, for 3 to 5 minutes, or until the chicken is ready. Stirring occasionally.
- Serve with cauliflower rice.

Fajitas
Time: 1 hour and 30 Mins, Serves: 6, Skill: Medium

Ingredients
- Dry cilantro (1/2 tsp)
- Lettuce wraps (4)
- Vegetable spray
- Vegetable oil (2 tbsp)
- Raw chicken strips (1 1/2 lb.), peeled and deveined
- Chili powder (2 tsp)
- Cumin (1/2 tsp)
- Lemon or lime juice (2 tbsp)
- Green and red pepper (1/4), sliced lengthwise
- White onion (1/2), sliced lengthwise

Instructions
- Preheat the oven to 300°F.
- Heat the vegetable oil in a non-stick pan over medium heat.
- Add the seasonings, lemon or lime juice, and chicken; simmer for 5 to 10 minutes, until meat is tender.
- In a pan, roast the onion and pepper for 1 to 2 minutes.
- Take it off the heat and add the coriander.
- Spoon the mix into each wrap, fold as desired and serve.

Seafood and Fish Recipes

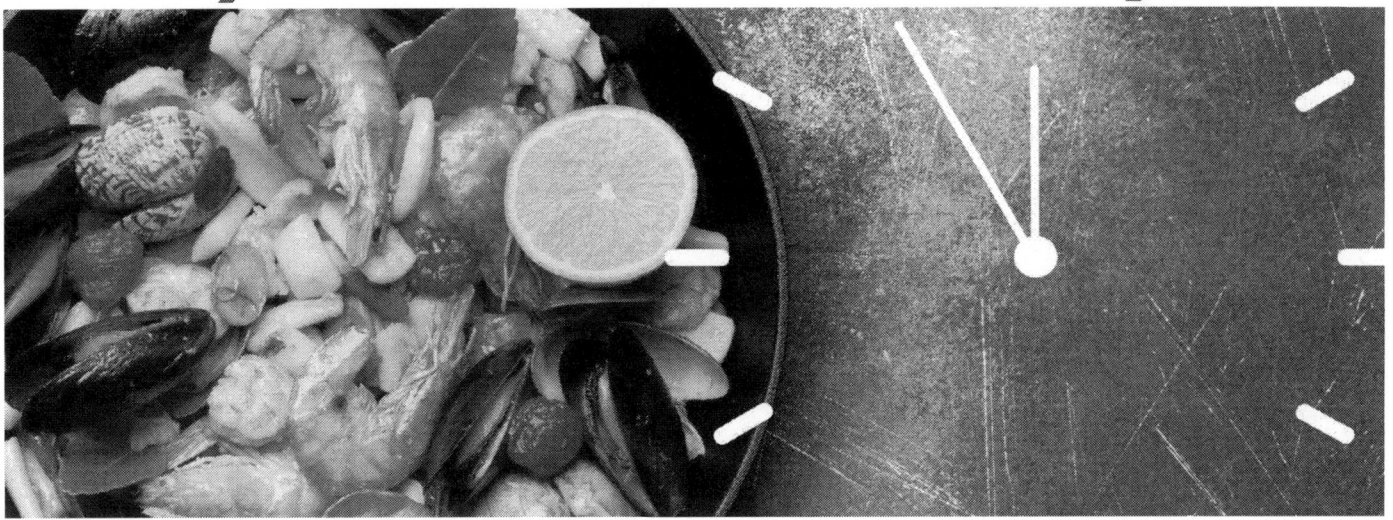

Refer to the end of the book for the conversion chart.

Grilled Trout
Time: 1 hour and 20 Mins, Serves: 2, Skill: Medium

Ingredients
- Lemon pepper (1 tsp), salt free
- Paprika (1/2 tsp)
- Rainbow trout fillets (2 lb.)
- Salt (1/2 tsp)
- Cooking oil (1 tbsp)

Instructions
- Preheat the grill to medium-high.
- Generously oil all sides of the trout fillets. Combine the spices in a bowl. Both fillets should be vigorously rubbed in the spices.
- Place the seasoned trout fillets on the preheated grill, skin side down. Grill for 4 minutes.
- Cook, flipping the fillets halfway through, for 3 to 5 minutes, or until the fish flakes easily with a fork.

Baked Salmon
Time: 1 hour and 5 Mins, Serves: 4, Skill: Easy

Ingredients
- Canned pimento (1/4 cup)
- Olive-oil based Mayonnaise (1/2 cup)
- Salmon (14 oz.), no salt, drained
- Onion (2/3 cup), chopped
- Ground flaxseed (1/4 cup)
- Green pepper (1/4 cup), diced
- Grated parmesan cheese (2 tsp)
- Non-stick cooking spray

Instructions
- Preheat the oven to 347 °F.
- Spray a baking tray with nonstick cooking spray.
- Combine the onion, mayonnaise, salmon, pimento, and pepper in a mixing bowl.
- Fill a baking jar halfway with the salmon mixture. On top, sprinkle ground flaxseed and Parmesan cheese.
- Bake for 20 minutes, or until the topping is light brown (or until completely heated).

Coconut Fish Dream
Time: 40 Mins, Serves: 4, Skill: Easy

Ingredients
- Turmeric (1/2 tbsp), ground
- Cod fillet (450g), cut into large chunks without skin
- Onion (1), chopped and grated
- Coconut milk (300 ml or 1/2-pint), unsweetened
- Garam masala (1/4 tsp)
- Cumin seeds (1 tbsp)
- Olive oil/Margarine (3 tsp), low salt
- Vegetable oil (1 tbsp)
- Green chilies (3), chopped
- Red chili powder (1/2 tbsp)
- Coriander (2 handfuls), chopped

Instructions
- Heat the oil and margarine/butter in a saucepan over low heat.
- Add the onion and cumin seeds, and cook until the onion is tender. Add the green chilies, chili powder, and ground turmeric. Mix together thoroughly.
- Once the sauce is vivid and the oil has spread, add a pinch of garam masala and whisk in the coconut milk. Add the cod and cook for a further 12-15 minutes.
- Garnish with a sprinkling of coriander before eating.
- Serve with rice and a spoonful of green salad.

Broiled Garlic Shrimp
Time: 1 hour, Serves: 4, Skill: Medium

Ingredients
- Pepper (1/8 teaspoon)
- Margarine (1/2 cup), unsalted, melted
- Lemon juice (2 tsp)
- Shrimp in shells (1 lb.)
- Fresh parsley (1 tbsp), chopped
- Onion (2 tbsp), chopped
- Garlic clove (1), minced

Instructions
- Preheat the broiler in the oven. Wash, dry, and peel the shrimp. Combine the margarine, lemon juice, onion, garlic, and pepper in a baking dish.
- Add the shrimp and cover with a lid.
- Cook for 5 minutes under the broiler. Broil for another 5 minutes on the other side.
- Serve on a tray with the pan juices diluted. Serve with a parsley garnish.

Shrimp Fajitas
Time: 45 Mins, Serves: 2, Skill: Easy

Ingredients
- Vegetable oil (2 tbsp)
- Dry cilantro (1/2 tsp)
- Lettuce wraps (4)
- Vegetable spray
- Raw shrimp (1 1/2 lb.), peeled and deveined
- Chili powder (2 tsp)
- Cumin (1/2 tsp)
- Lemon or lime juice (2 tbsp)
- Green and red pepper (1/4), sliced lengthwise
- White onion (1/2), sliced lengthwise

Instructions
- Preheat the oven to 300°F.
- In a nonstick tray, heat the vegetable oil over low heat.
- Add the seasonings, lemon or lime juice, and shrimps. Cook for 5 to 10 minutes, or until tender.
- Add the onion and pepper and roast for 1 to 2 minutes.
- Remove the pan from the heat and stir in the coriander.
- Bake the tortillas after arranging them on the foil. Cook for a maximum of 10 minutes.
- Divide the mixture among the tortillas, wrap them and serve.

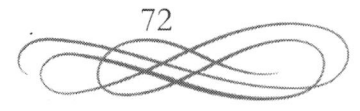

Spanish Paella

Time: 1 hour 15 Mins, Serves: 2, Skill: Medium

Ingredients
- Red bell pepper (1/3 cup), chopped
- Green onion (1/3 cup), sliced
- Garlic cloves 2, minced
- Pepper (1/4 tsp)
- Chicken breast (1/2 lb.), boneless and skinless, cut into 1/2-inch piece
- Water (1/4 cup)
- Chicken broth (10-1/2-oz can), low in salt
- Medium-size shrimp (1/2 lb.), peeled & cleaned
- Frozen green peas (1/2 cup)
- Ground saffron (a dash)
- Cauliflower rice (1 cup), uncooked

Instructions
- In a two-quart casserole dish, combine the first three ingredients and cover with the lid. Microwave for 4 to 5 minutes on heavy.
- Combine the shrimp and the remaining ingredients in the casserole dish. Cover and cook for 3 and 1/2 to 4 1/2 minutes on warm, or until the shrimp turns pink.
- Add the rice and mix thoroughly. Cook for 5 minutes, or until the rice is tender.

Shrimp Salad

Time: 1 hour and 20 Mins, Serves: 3, Skill: Hard

Ingredients
- Green pepper (1 tbsp), chopped
- Onion (1 tbsp), chopped
- Tabasco or hot sauce (1/8 tbsp)
- Mayonnaise (2 tbsp), low fat
- Chili powder (1/2 tbsp)
- Lemon juice (1 tbsp)
- Shrimp (1 lb.), chopped, boiled, & deveined
- Hard-boiled egg (1), chopped
- Lettuce, shredded or chopped (optional)
- Celery (1 tbsp), chopped
- Mustard dry (1/2 tbsp)

Instructions
- In a mixing bowl, combine all ingredients except the lettuce and thoroughly blend.
- Chill in the refrigerator for 30 minutes before serving.
- Serve in a lettuce-covered dish or on a sandwich.

Seafood Croquettes

Time: 1 hour and 30 Mins, Serves: 4, Skill: Hard

Ingredients
- Water-packed salmon or tuna (1 can 14.75-oz.)
- Almond flour or almond flour Cracker crumbs (1/2 cup), unsalted
- Cooking spray or vegetable oil (1) tbsp
- Crab meat (1 lb.), frozen or fresh
- Regular mayonnaise (1/4 cup)
- Egg whites (2)
- Ground mustard (1/2 tbsp)
- Onion (1/4 cup), chopped
- Lemon juice (2 tbsp), optional
- Black pepper (1/2 tbsp)

Instructions
- Drain the canned salmon or tuna.
- In a medium bowl, mix all the ingredients except the oil. Ensuring you mix it rigorously.
- Split the mixture into eight balls and flatten each one to produce patties.
- Heat the vegetable oil in a skillet.
- Slowly lower the patties into the boiling oil.
- Softly brown the patties on both sides. If the patties are fried in grease, drain them on paper towels when cooked.
- Bake the patties instead of frying for a healthier version.

Salmon Salad
Time: 30 Mins, Serves: 2, Skill: Easy

Ingredients
- Ken's Honey Mustard Dipping Sauce (2 tbsp), low sugar
- Celery (1/4 cup), chopped
- Red onion (1/4 cup), chopped
- Red pepper (1/4 cup), chopped
- Canned salmon (12 oz.), low sodium

Instructions
- Chop the celery, red pepper & red onion into small bits.
- Mix it with honey mustard and salmon and serve.

Crab Cakes
Time: 30 Mins, Serves: 4, Skill: Easy

Ingredients
- Garlic powder (1 tsp)
- Egg (1), egg substitute or egg white optional
- Green or red pepper (1/3 cup), finely chopped
- Almond flour crackers (1/3 cup), low sodium
- Mayonnaise (1/4 cup), reduced-fat
- Dry mustard (1 tbsp)
- Crushed red pepper or black pepper (1 tsp)
- Lemon juice (2 tbsp)
- Vegetable oil (2 tbsp)

Instructions
- In a mixing bowl, combine all the ingredients.
- Shape patties by dividing the mixture into 6 spheres.
- Heat the vegetable oil in a medium-hot pan or a 347 °F oven.
- In a hot pan, cook the patties for 4 to 5 minutes.
- Serve immediately.

Salad Recipes

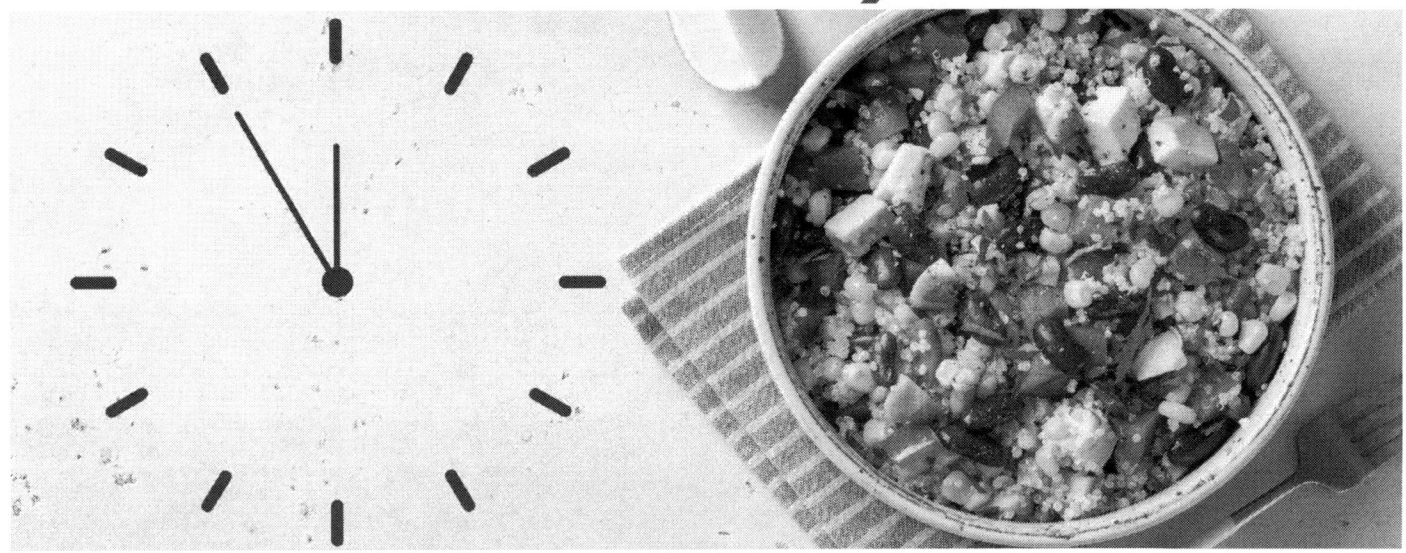

Refer to the end of the book for the conversion chart.

Crunchy Cauliflower Salad
Time: 45 Mins, Serves: 8, Skill: Easy

Ingredients
- Water (2 cups)
- Cucumbers (1/2 cup), seeded and diced
- Cauliflower rice (1 cup), steamed
- Green onions (3), chopped
- Fresh mint (1/4 cup), chopped
- Lemon rind (1 tbsp), zest
- Olive oil (4 tbsp)
- Parmesan cheese (1/4 cup), low sodium, grated
- Head Boston or Bibb lettuce (1/2)
- Leaf parsley (1/2 cup), chopped
- Lemon juice (2 tbsp)

Instructions
- Steam cauliflower rice for 20 minutes in a pot, add 1 cup water, over medium-high heat, stirring periodically.. Allow a couple of minutes of cooking before fluffing with a fork.
- Combine the mint, parsley, zest, lemon juice, and olive oil with cucumbers, and onions. Toss the rice into the blend (cooled).
- Cover lettuce cups halfway with the mixture and top with parmesan cheese.

Buttermilk Herb Ranch Dressing
Time: 40 Mins, Serves: 2, Skill: Easy

Ingredients
- Almond Milk (1/2 cup)
- Vinegar (2 tbsp)
- Fresh chives (1 tbsp), chopped
- Dill (1 tbsp)
- Greek yogurt (1/2 cup)
- Oregano Leaves (1 tbsp), chopped
- Garlic powder (1/4 tsp)

Instructions
- Combine the mayonnaise, milk, and vinegar in a medium mixing cup.
- Add 1/4 teaspoon of garlic powder, fresh chives, oregano leaves, and dill.
- Come them together.

- Refrigerate for at least 1 hour to allow flavors to develop.
- To serve, drizzle the dressing on top of a salad.

Green Beans Salad

Time: 30 Mins, Serves: 4, Skill: Easy

Ingredients

- Oil (1 tbsp)
- Lemon juice (1/2)
- Black pepper, freshly ground, to taste
- Water (12 cups)
- Green beans (1 1/2 lb.), rinsed and ends trimmed

Sauce:

- Stevia (1 tbsp)
- Water (1 tbsp)
- Garlic clove (1 large), minced
- Oil (1 tsp)

Instructions

- Get the stockpot's water to a low boil and add the beans. Cook for 3 minutes, or until the beans are light green in color. Be cautious not to overcook them.
- Remove and rinse the beans for 1 minute in cold water. Place the dried beans in a big mixing bowl after they have cooled.
- To create a sauce, blend stevia, garlic, water, and 1 teaspoon of oil in a mixing cup.
- Heat 1 tablespoon of oil in a wide skillet over low heat. Swirl the beans in the oil. Continue to stir for about 3 minutes after adding the sauce. Green beans that are finished will be bright green and crisp-tender.
- Switch to a serving bowl.
- Now add some pepper (black) and lime juice to enhance the taste.
- Serve and enjoy.

Violet, Green Salad

Time: 35 Mins, Serves: 4, Skill: Easy

Ingredients

- Frozen peas (1 cup)
- Pear (1)
- Goat cheese (3 oz)
- Chive flowers, violets, or edible flowers (1 oz)
- Plain or Greek plain yogurt (1/4 cup)
- Pomegranate molasses (1/4 cup), sugar free
- Spring greens (4 cups)
- Cucumber (1)
- Lemon juice (2 tbsp)
- Fresh parsley (1/4 cup)
- Nuts (1/4 cup), optional
- Olive oil (1/2 cup)
- Mustard (1 tsp)
- Allspice (1 pinch)

Instructions

- Cut the greens into bite-sized sections.
- Cucumbers can be split into discs, then quartered.
- To use frozen peas, split the pods in thirds and thaw at room temperature for around half an hour.
- In a mixing dish, combine the diced pear and greens.
- If you have some remaining goat cheese, blend it with the chives and break it into 1/2-inch pieces.
- Combine the yogurt, lemon juice, molasses, parsley, allspice, olive oil, and mustard in a food processor or mixer.
- In a big mixing dish, combine the salad and the dressing.
- For a dazzling show, scatter goat cheese, spices, and nuts around the surface.

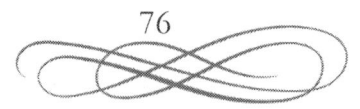

Cabbage with Strawberries
Time: 30 Mins, Serves: 6, Skill: Easy

Ingredients
- Olive or vegetable oil (2 tbsp)
- Cider vinegar (1/4 cup)
- Stevia (2 tbsp)
- Fresh Strawberries (1 cup)
- Green Cabbage (1 small)
- Onion (1), coarsely chopped

Instructions
- Sauté the onion in the oil in a wide skillet until softened (nearly 5 minutes).
- Add the vinegar, cinnamon, and sugar; combine the strawberries and cabbage.
- Bring to a boil, then reduce to low heat, cover, and simmer until the cabbage wilts, around 15 minutes.

Creamy Fruit Salad
Time: 25 Mins, Serves: 4, Skill: Easy

Ingredients
- Peaches (2 medium), diced
- Plain Greek yogurt (1 cup)
- Cinnamon (1/2 tsp), add stevia (1 tsp) (cinnamon-stevia)
- Lemon (1), juiced
- Strawberries (1 cup), cut in quarters, lengthwise
- Dried cranberries (1 cup)

Instructions
- In a medium mixing cup, combine all the berries.
- In a small cup, combine the yogurt, lemon juice, and cinnamon stevia mixture. To create a full mix, add all the ingredients in a blender.
- Toss the fruit and yogurt mixture together. Combine the products, sample, and change the seasoning as required.
- Refrigerated leftovers can be stored for up to 2 days.

Broccoli Rice Salad
Time: 1 hour 20 Mins, Serves: 8, Skill: Medium

Ingredients
- Olive oil (1 tbsp)
- Walnuts (2/3 cup), chopped
- Celery rib (4 inches), sliced
- Scallions (4), thinly sliced
- Fresh Cranberries (2/3 cup)
- Red apple (1 medium), semi-tart, cored and diced
- Pomegranate seeds (1/2 cup)
- Broccoli rice (1 cup)
- Water (2 cups)
- Lemon zest (1/2 tbsp)
- Lemon juice (3 tbsp)
- Black pepper, freshly ground, to taste
- Olive oil (1/3 cup)
- Sea salt (1/2 tsp)

Instructions
- In a medium saucepan, mix broccoli rice with oil, water, and salt if appropriate. Carry to a boil, then drop to low heat to sustain a gentle simmer.
- Cook for 10 minutes, or until the liquid has evaporated.
- In a large mixing cup, combine the walnuts, scallions, cranberries, celery, apples, pomegranate seeds, and lemon zest.
- In a container with a tight-fitting cap, mix the lemon juice, olive oil, and pepper and shake vigorously.
- Toss the apple mixture with half of the dressing and toss well.
- Set the rice aside to cool until it's just mildly moist.
- Serve with the leftover dressing and the fruit combination in a cup or on a lettuce bed at room temperature.

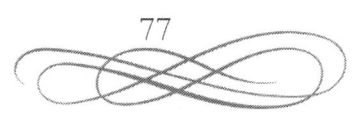

Shrimp Salad with Cucumber Mint
Time: 30 Mins, Serves: 6, Skill: Easy

Ingredients
- Fresh mint leaves (1 cup)
- Lemon juice (2 tbsp)
- Olive oil (3 tbsp)
- Cucumber (1/2), seeded, diced
- Lemon zest (1)
- Med shrimp (2 lb.), cleaned
- Pepper, to taste

Instructions
- Blanch the shrimp for 3 minutes in boiling water, then drain and put aside.
- In a blender or food processor, combine the mint and lemon juice and pulse to coarsely chop the mint.
- Drizzle in the olive oil after pureeing the mint until it is finely sliced.
- Combine the shrimp, mint blend, cucumber, zest, and pepper in a bowl and serve.

Fire and Ice Watermelon Salsa
Time: 25 Mins, Serves: 6, Skill: Easy

Ingredients
- Green bell pepper (1 cup), chopped
- Lime juice (2 tbsp)
- Cilantro (1 tbsp), chopped
- Green onion (1 tbsp), chopped
- Jalapeño (2 meds), seeded and minced
- Garlic clove (1), crushed
- Watermelon (2 cups), chopped

Instructions
- In a large mixing bowl, combine all the ingredients and mix thoroughly.
- Chill for at least an hour before serving.
- Serve with chicken or seafood as a sauce or a dip.

Riced Cauliflower Salad
Time: 35 Mins, Serves: 6, Skill: Easy

Ingredients
- Pomegranate seeds (1/2 cup)
- Almonds (1/2 cup), sliced or chopped
- Mint (1/2 cup), chopped
- Black beans (1 cup)
- Cranberries (1/2 cup), dried, unsweetened
- Cauliflower (4 1/2 cups), riced
- Lemon (1), zested
- Lemons (2), juiced
- Olive oil (1/4 cup)

Instructions
- Cut the core and leaves from the cauliflower florets and grate them on the wide whole side of a box grater.
- In a big salad bowl, position the riced cauliflower.
- Toss in the pomegranate, mint, almonds, cranberries, black beans, and lemon zest.
- Toss the salad with lemon juice and olive oil, gently mixing all ingredients.
- Serve with crisp bread or as a side salad for lunch.

Fruity Chicken Salad
Time: 35 Mins, Serves: 8, Skill: Easy

Ingredients
- Apple (1), cubed
- Cranberries (3/4 cup)
- Greek yogurt (1/2 cup)
- Mayonnaise (1/4 cup), low-fat
- Rice vinegar (1 tsp), unseason
- Stevia (2 tsp)
- Chicken breasts (2 cups), cooked
- Almonds (1 cup), sliced
- Celery stalk (1), chopped
- Green onion (1), chopped
- Berries (2 cups)
- Chinese five-spice blend (1/2 tsp)

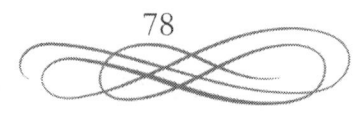

Instructions

- Combine the chicken, celery, green onion, almonds, berries, apples, and cranberries in a big mixing bowl.
- Blend the sour cream, rice vinegar, mayonnaise, stevia, and Chinese 5-Spice in a separate cup.
- In a mixing bowl, combine the chicken and the dressing.

Lemon Curry Chicken Salad
Time: 25 Mins, Serves: 4, Skill: Easy

Ingredient

- Olive oil (1/4 cup)
- Celery (1/2 cup), sliced
- Fresh lemon juice (1/4 cup), add stevia (1 tsp)
- Ground ginger (1/4 tsp)
- Curry powder (1/4 tsp)
- Garlic powder (1/8 tsp)
- Chicken (1 1/2 cups), cooked and diced
- Berries (1 1/2 cups)

Instructions

- Combine the lemon mixture, oil, and spices in a big mixing cup.
- Gently toss in the remaining ingredients.
- Serve after 1 hour marinating.

Snacks & Side Recipes

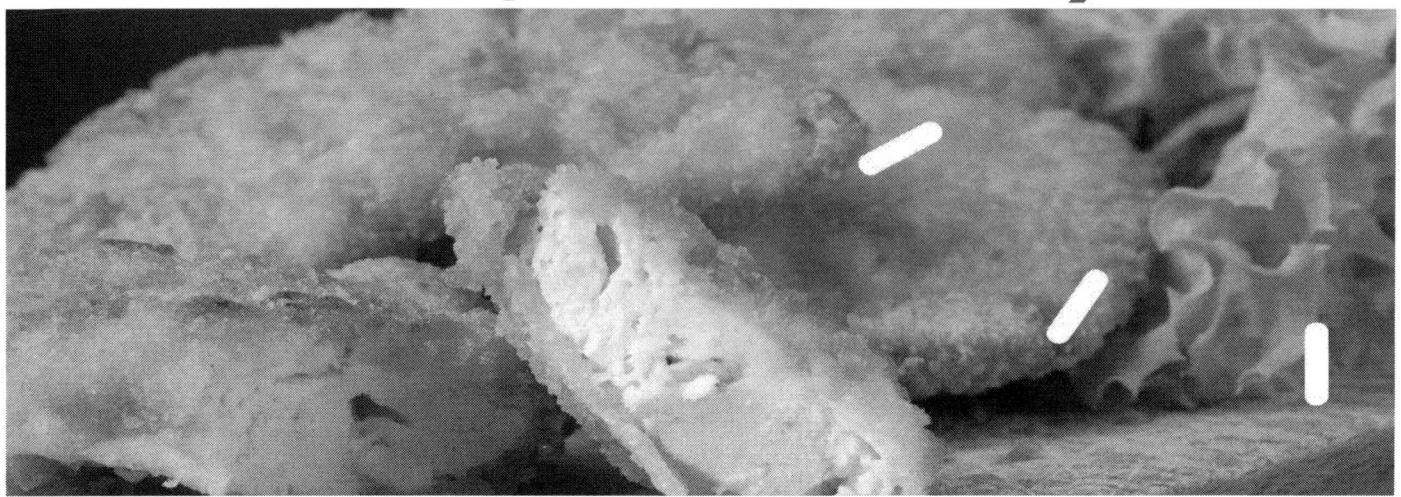

Refer to the end of the book for the conversion chart.

Anytime Energy Bars
Time: 1 hour and 15 Mins, Serves: 8, Skill: Hard

Ingredients
- Mixed nuts and seeds (1 cup)
- Eggs (3 large)
- Applesauce (1/3 cup), sugar-free
- Stevia (3 tbsp)
- Cinnamon (1/2 tsp), ground
- Peanuts (3 tbsp), unsalted, chopped
- Dark small chocolate chips (1/4 cup), sugar free
- Coconut (1/3 cup), shredded

Instructions
- Preheat the oven to 325 °F and spray a 9x9-inch baking pan with cooking oil.
- Combine the nuts and seeds, chocolate chips, cinnamon, peanuts, and coconut in a large mixing cup.
- In a small mixing cup, whisk the eggs. Add stevia and applesauce.
- In a large mixing cup, completely blend the egg and oat mixture.
- Place the mixture evenly onto the rim of the greased pan.
- Cooking time is 40 minutes. Allow it to cool completely before cutting it into bars.

Easy baked pears
Time: 45 Mins, Serves: 4, Skill: Easy

Ingredients
- Cinnamon (1/2 tsp), ground
- Monk fruit (4 tbsp)
- Ginger biscuits (8)
- Ripe pears (4)
- Crème Fraiche (4 level tbsp), reduced-fat

Instructions
- To start, preheat the oven to 374 °F.
- Split each pear in 1/2. Using a teaspoon, scrape out the cores. In the center of each make a dip. Place them, sliced side up, on the baking sheet.
- Sprinkle monk fruit over the top and season with cinnamon.
- Roast the pears for 10 to 15 mins, or until tender. Crush some biscuits of ginger and sprinkle them on top, and serve along with a cream fraiche (spoonful).

Sunshine Carrots
Time: 20 Mins, Serves: 4, Skill: Easy

Ingredients
- Carrots (3 cups), sliced
- Parsley (1 tsp), chopped, fresh, for garnish
- Monk fruit (1 tbsp)
- Lemon juice (1 tbsp)
- Lemon peel (1/4 tsp), grated
- Margarine (2 tbsp)

Instructions
- Cook the carrots until soft in boiling water; rinse well.
- In a mixing cup, combine the butter, Monk fruit, lemon juice, margarine, and lemon peel.

Southern-fried okra
Time: 45 Mins, Serves: 6, Skill: Easy

Ingredients
- Salt (1/8 tsp)
- Avocado oil (1/3 cup)
- Almond flour (1/2 cup)
- Cayenne pepper (1/4 tbsp)
- Black pepper (1/4 tbsp)
- Almond Milk (2 tbsp)
- Egg (1)
- Coconut Flour (1/2 cup)
- Okra (3 cups), sliced

Instructions
- Combine the black pepper, flour, salt, cayenne pepper, and almond flour and coconut flour in a mixing dish.
- In a separate dish, mix the almond milk and egg.
- Drop the okra parts into the egg mixture, then roll them in the flour mixture before putting them aside.
- In a pan, heat sunflower oil and fry coated okra bits for 2 minutes.
- Or, bake the fried bits for 3 minutes at 300°F in a preheated oven.

Champ – Side Dish Cauliflower Mash
Time: 35 Mins, Serves: 2, Skill: Easy

Ingredients
- Cauliflower mash (600 g)
- Black pepper, ground
- Onions (2), chopped
- Almond Milk (1-2 tbsp)

Instructions
- In a big saucepan of water, boil the cauliflower until soft.
- Mash the cauliflower once you have added the black pepper, milk, and spring onions.

Slovakian Sauerkraut and Zucchini Noodles
Time: 55 Mins, Serves: 5, Skill: Easy

Ingredients
- Zucchini noodles (6 oz.)
- Sauerkraut (4 oz.), drained
- Black pepper (1/2 tsp), ground
- Butter (2 tbsp), unsalted
- Onion (1/2 small/35g), diced
- Dill (1 tbsp), fresh, chopped

Instructions
- Melt one tablespoon of butter over medium heat in a large skillet
- Add the onions. Cook, stirring regularly, until the onions are smooth and transparent, around 5 minutes.
- Put a broad pot halfway full of water to a boil.
- Add the zucchini noodles to the boiling broth for 10 minutes or until tender.
- Add the sauerkraut and 1/2 tablespoon more butter to the fried onions. Since thoroughly blending, boil for 3 minutes.
- Combine the noodles, sauerkraut, and the remaining 1/2 tablespoon of butter in the same pan. Blend well after seasoning with black pepper.
- Garnish with dill on top. You should serve it with a side salad.

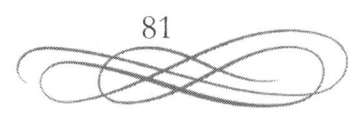

Deviled Eggs
Time: 45 Mins, Serves: 8, Skill: Easy

Ingredients
- Cider vinegar (1 tsp)
- Stevia (1 tsp)
- Yellow mustard (1 tsp)
- Onion powder (1/2 tsp)
- Eggs (6), hard-boiled
- Mayonnaise (2 tbsp), low-fat

Instructions
- Halve the eggs and set aside the whites and yolks separately.
- In a shallow bowl, mash the yolks with a fork. Add the mayonnaise, vinegar, onion powder, stevia, and mustard. Blend until fully smooth.
- Place the mixture in a piping bag and pipe it into the egg white halves.
- If necessary, garnish with paprika. Refrigerate before serving.

Taco Seasoning
Time: 35 Mins, Serves: 5, Skill: Easy

Ingredients
- Onion powder (1 tbsp)
- Oregano (1 tsp), dried
- Garlic powder (1 tsp)
- Red pepper (1 tsp), crushed
- Cinnamon (1/2 tsp)
- Chili powder (1/4 cup)
- Cumin (1 tbsp), ground

Instructions
- In an airtight jar, combine all the ingredients and store until usage.

Swiss Chard Crostini
Time: 35 Mins, Serves: 10, Skill: Easy

Ingredients
- Olive oil (2 tbsp)
- Garlic cloves (3)
- Water (3 tbsp)
- Baguette or low-carb bread (1/2), sliced into 10, ½-inch slices
- Swiss chard (1/2 bunch/6 oz.)
- Ricotta cheese (1/2 cup)

Instructions
- Toast the baguette slices until finely browned in a toaster oven or a standard oven at 300°F.
- Extract the Swiss chard's roots. To build a leaf mound, arrange the leaves in four layers. Roll horizontally and slice into the rolls to create leaf ribbons.
- Continue until all the leaves are trimmed.
- Melt the olive oil in a large skillet over medium heat. For 2 minutes, stirring halfway through, roast the Swiss chard and garlic. Reduce to a low heat and place in boiling water. Cook until the chard is soft but still has a light green color.
- Position the toasted baguette slices on a serving tray to assemble. Spread a thin layer of ricotta on each piece. Place the cooked chard on top of the ricotta toast with tongs. Serve as a snack or an appetizer.

Spiced Pepitas
Time: 40 Mins, Serves: 8, Skill: Easy

Ingredients
- Monk fruit (1 tbsp)
- Cumin seed (1 tsp), grounded
- Butter (1 1/2 tbsp), unsalted
- Pepitas (1 1/2 cups)

Instructions
- In a skillet over low heat, melt the butter, then stir in monk fruit and cumin until well combined.
- To fairly spread the pepitas, apply them and combine for 1 to 2 minutes.
- Remove the pan from the heat and set it aside to cool.
- Any serving may be enjoyed alone, or with a slice of fruit or cheese as a snack.

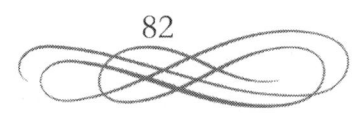

Meat Recipes

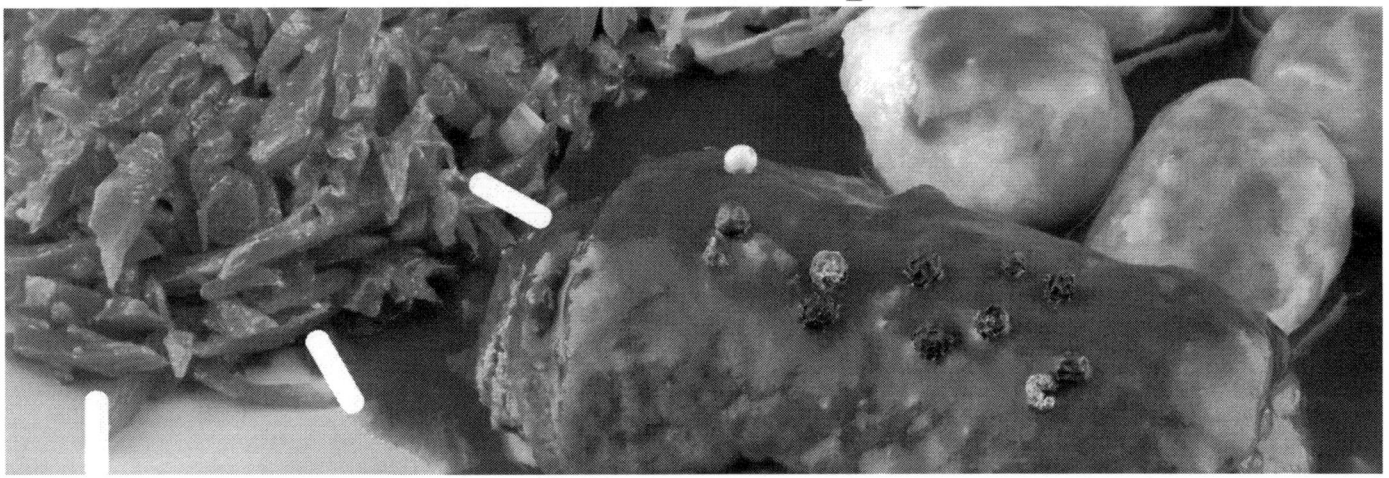

Refer to the end of the book for the conversion chart.

Beef Curry
Time: 3 hours, Serves: 4, Skill: Hard

Ingredients
- Avocado oil (5 tbsp)
- Beef with bone (1-1/2 lb.), small
- Whole cumin seeds (3/4 tsp)
- Salt (3/4 tsp)
- Bay leaves (2)
- Whole peppercorns (1/4 tsp)
- Cayenne pepper (1-1/2 tsp)
- Cinnamon stick (1)
- Garam masala (1/2 tsp)
- Tomato (1 medium)
- Garlic cloves (2)
- Onions (2 medium)
- Ginger root (1" cube)

Instructions
- Peel and chop the tomato. Mince the garlic, pepper, and ginger root.
- Heat the oil in a large, thick pot over medium-high heat. Add the cumin seeds, bay leaves, cinnamon sticks, and peppercorns, stirring occasionally.
- Add the garlic, ginger, and onion, and cook until brown specks appear on the onion.
- Add the beef, cabbage, cayenne pepper, flour, and a quarter cup of water to the pan and blend well. Bring to a low simmer, stirring regularly.
- Cover the pan, lower the heat to low, and simmer for 45 minutes, or until the beef is tender and juicy. Continue to stir during the cooking period.
- Remove the cover and maintain a low heat. To minimize the amount of oil used, season with garam masala and fry, stirring periodically, for around 5 minutes.

Beef Casserole
Time: 40 Mins, Serves: 2, Skill: Easy

Ingredients
- Salt (1/4 tsp)
- Fresh parsley (1 tbsp), chopped
- Lean beef (500g)
- Water (350ml)
- Onion (1 medium), chopped
- Olive oil (1 tbsp)

- Zucchini (2 medium), peeled and sliced
- White pepper (1/4 tsp)

Instructions

- Fry the onion in a limited volume of oil.
- Add the beef and cook until it is browned.
- Then add some water and cook until the beef is tender.
- Add the zucchini and onions to the meat and proceed to cook until the vegetables and the meat are cooked through.
- Apply salt, pepper, and finely chopped parsley to taste.

Hawaiian-Style Slow-Cooked Beef
Time: 6 Hours, Serves: 4, Skill: Hard

Ingredients

- Onion powder (1 tsp)
- Paprika (1/2 tsp)
- Organic liquid smoke (2 tbsp)
- Boneless Beef (4 lb.)
- Black pepper (1/2 tsp), freshly ground
- Pickled or radishes red onions (optional garnish)
- Garlic powder (1/2 tsp)

Instructions

- In a bag, add black pepper, paprika, garlic powder, and onion.
- Rub the beef with the flavoring paste all over. In a slow cooker or a cooker, position the beef. Sprinkle with liquid smoke.
- Pour sufficient water into the crock-pot or slow cooker to fill it to a depth of 14–12 inches. Cook for 4–5 hours on high pressure.
- Shred the beef with two forks after extracting it from the cooker.
- Serve it warm.

Fiesta Lime Tacos
Time: 14 Mins, Serves: 12, Skill: Easy

Ingredients

- Water (3/4 cup)
- Lean ground beef or turkey (1 lb.)
- Mrs. Dash Fiesta Lime Seasoning Blend (4 tbsp), additive sugar free
- Taco shells (12), or lettuce wraps

Instructions

- Brown the ground beef in a large skillet over medium-high heat.
- Get rid of the excess fat.
- Add the water and Mrs. Dash Fiesta Lime Seasoning Mixture.
- Bring the water to a boil. Reduce the heat to low and simmer, stirring occasionally, for 5 minutes.
- Scoop the meat mixture into taco shells or lettuce wraps that are already soft. If chosen, serve with additional toppings.

Seasoned Pork Chops
Time: 1 hour and 10 Mins, Serves: 3, Skill: Hard

Ingredients

- Lean pork chops (4 x 4-ounce), fat removed
- Vegetable oil (2 tbsp)
- Thyme (1/2 tbsp)
- Almond flour (1/4 cup)
- Black pepper (1 tsp)
- Sage (1/2 tbsp)

Instructions

- Preheat the oven to 350 °F.
- Spray the skillet with cooking spray.
- In a mixing dish, combine the almond flour, sage, black pepper, and thyme.
- Dredge the chops in the almond flour mix and drop them in the baking tray with the oil.
- Put it in the oven for about 40 minutes, or until it is juicy on all sides.

Parsley Burger
Time: 1 hour and 10 Mins, Serves: 1, Skill: Medium

Ingredients

- Oregano (1/4 tbsp)

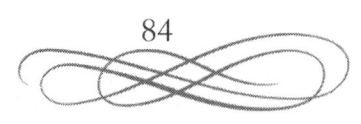

- Slender organic ground turkey or grass-fed beef (1 lb.)
- Thyme (1/4 tbsp), ground
- Lemon juice (1 tbsp)
- Black pepper (1/4 tbsp)
- Parsley flakes (1 tbsp)

Instructions
- Gently blend all the ingredients in a large mixing cup.
- Shape into four small patties, each around 3/4 inches in diameter.
- Put in a skillet or broiler pan that has been finely greased.
- Broil for 10 to 15 minutes after turning, about 3" from the flame.

Easy Beef Burgers
Time: 1 hour 10 Mins, Serves: 2, Skill: Medium

Ingredients
- Dried mixed herbs (a pinch)
- Onion (1), chopped
- Black pepper
- Grass-fed Beef or pork (500 g), low in fat, minced

Instruction:
- Ready the grill or barbecue by preheating it. Combine all the ingredients in a big mixing cup.
- Using clean, damp hands, split it into 8 small or 4 large patties. Cut the beef into flattish rounds of similar depth to ensure even and detailed cooking.
- Cook for 5 to 10 minutes on either side on the grill.
- Both the inside and outside of the burgers must be brown. Serve on pita bread or a sandwich bun with sliced lettuce and a spoonful of mayonnaise, tomato sauce, or vinegar.

Tortilla Beef Rollups
Time: 25 Mins, Serves: 2, Skill: Easy

Ingredients
- Romaine lettuce leaves (2)
- Roast beef (5 oz.), cooked
- Red onion (1/4 cup), chopped
- Cucumber (8 slices)
- Low-carb tortilla (2), 6" size
- Red/Green or Yellow bell pepper (1/4), cut in strips
- Cream cheese (2 tbsp), whipped
- Herb seasoning blend (1 tbsp)

Instructions
- Place the tortillas on a plate and spread cream cheese on top.
- Split the products in half to produce two tortillas. On each tortilla, layer the roast beef, pepper strips, red onion, cucumbers, & lettuce.
- Season with a pinch of salt and pepper.
- Fold tortillas.
- Serve each tortilla whole or cut into 4 parts.

Jamaican Beef Patties
Time: 1 hour and 20 Mins, Serves: 2, Skill: Medium

Ingredients
- Garlic clove (1), chopped
- Fresh chili (1), minced
- Chili powder (1 tbsp.)
- Thyme (1/2 tbsp), dried
- Short crust pastry, almond-flour based crust (500g or 1 lb.), one packet
- Beef (200g or 8oz.), minced
- Pork rinds (4 tbsp)
- Onion (1 small), chopped
- Curry powder (1 tbsp)

Instruction:
- Preheat the oven to 400°F.
- Cook the chopped garlic and onion with the minced beef in a nonstick frying pan until the meat is nearly brown. Cook for 15 minutes

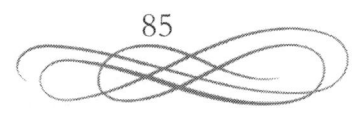

with the breadcrumbs and seasoning, covered, over a low flame. Using a colander or sieve, drain and remove any remaining liquid.
- On a saucer, roll out the pastry to make 6 circles.
- Divide the beef evenly among the pastry rings. To close the pastry, dampen the sides, cut it in half, and press the corners together. Rub it with milk and place it on a baking tray.
- Bake for 25-30 minutes, or until golden brown, in the center of the oven.

Chili Rice with Beef
Time: 50 Mins, Serves: 1, Skill: Easy

Ingredients
- Cauliflower Rice (2 cups), cooked
- Onion (1 cup), chopped
- Black pepper (1/8 tsp)
- Chili con carne seasoning powder (1 1/2 tsp), sugar free
- Sage (1/2 tsp)
- Ground beef (1 lb.), lean
- Vegetable oil (2 tbsp)

Instructions
- In a skillet, heat the oil and add the beef and onion. Fry until golden brown, stirring constantly.
- Apply fried rice and spices to the combination. S
- Remove the combination from the flames. Cover with a lid and set aside for 10-14 minutes.

Soup & Stew Recipes

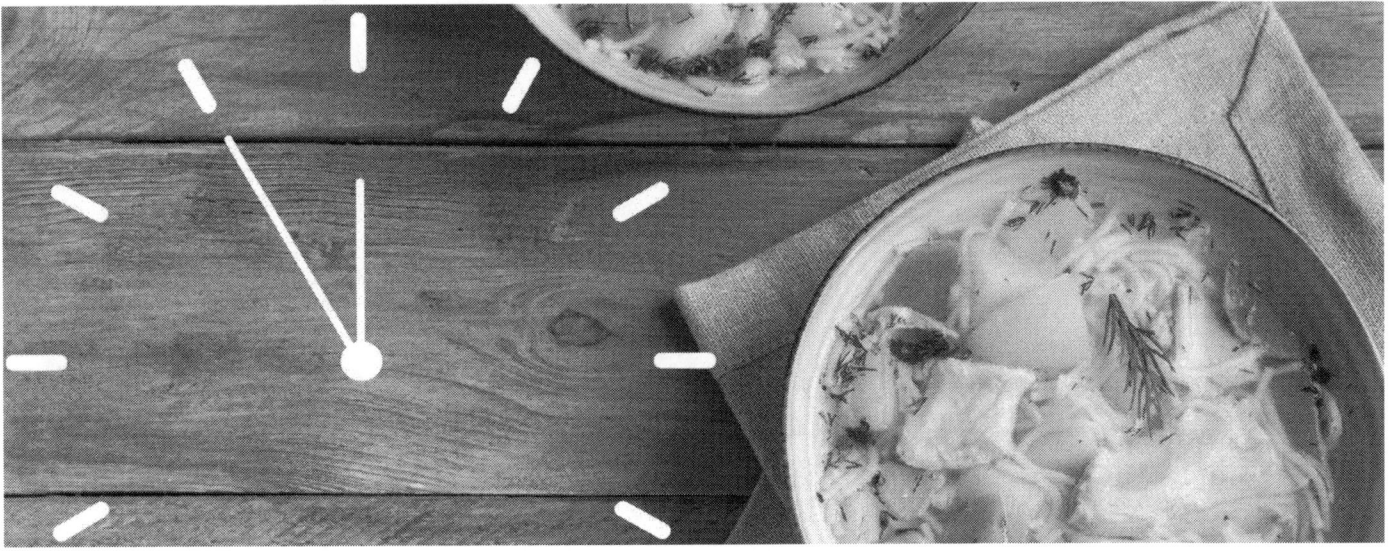

Refer to the end of the book for the conversion chart.

Thai Chicken Soup
Time: 50 Mins, Serves: 4, Skill: Easy

Ingredients
- Stevia (1 tbsp)
- Chili sauce/chili flakes (1 tsp)
- Lemongrass stalk (1), chopped
- Ginger (1"), sliced
- Lite coconut milk (1 can)
- White button mushrooms (10), quartered
- Red bell pepper (1), sliced
- Yellow onion (1/2), sliced
- Lime juice (2 tbsp)
- Chicken breast (1 lb.), or shrimp
- Simple Chicken Broth (4 cups), other low sodium broth
- Fish sauce (1/2 tbsp)

Instructions
- In a large pot coated with nonstick cooking oil, brown the shrimp or chicken until evenly browned.
- Add the broth, fish sauce, chili sauce, ginger, and lemongrass.
- Reduce the heat to medium-low and cook for 10 to 15 minutes, stirring periodically.
- Add the coconut milk, bell pepper, mushrooms, and onions. Simmer for 5 minutes.
- Lime juice can be added just before serving.

Cauliflower Rice Soup
Time: 1 hour and 5 Mins, Serves: 4, Skill: Medium

Ingredients
- Red onion (1 cup), diced small
- Garlic powder (1 1/2 tsp)
- Dried thyme (1/2 tsp)
- Pepper (1/4 tsp)
- Salt (1/2 tsp)
- Cauliflower rice (1/2 cup)
- Water (6 cups)
- Olive oil (1 tbsp)
- Celery (1/2 cup), sliced
- Kale (2 cups), stemmed & leaves chopped
- Parsley (1/4 cup), chopped

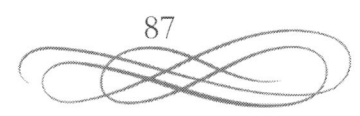

- Lemon juice (1 tbsp)

Instructions

- In a wide pot, heat the oil, then add the onions and celery and cook, stirring occasionally, for 3 to 4 minutes, or until slightly brown.
- Add the seasonings, garlic powder, salt, dried thyme, and pepper. Cook for about 30 seconds, or until fragrant, stirring constantly.
- Toast the cauliflower rice for at least 2 minutes after mixing it in.
- In the water, mix it together. Bring to a simmer, sealed, over high flame.
- Reduce heat to low and simmer for around 50 minutes, stirring regularly, until it starts to boil.
- Cook for another 5 minutes after adding the kale.
- Add the parsley and lemon juice. Pots may be used to prepare the soup.

Minestrone Soup
Time: 1 hour and 20 Mins, Serves: 4, Skill: Medium

Ingredients

- Onion (1/2 large), diced
- Garlic cloves (4), minced
- Italian seasoning (1 tsp)
- Black pepper (1/2 tsp)
- Vegetable stock (4 cups), no-salt-added
- Tomatoes (14.5 oz.), diced, no-salt-added, 1 can
- Mixed vegetables (10 oz.), frozen
- Olive oil (2 tbsp)
- Whole grain pasta (3 oz.)

Instructions

- Heat the liquid in a broad pot over medium-low heat. Cook the garlic, onion, pepper, and Italian seasoning, stirring occasionally. About 8 minutes.
- Allow the onions, mixed vegetables, and tomatoes to boil in the cooker. Cook until the dry pasta is just under al dente.
- Serve immediately.

Quick Mushroom Broth
Time: 40 Mins, Serves: 2, Skill: Easy

Ingredients

- Dried mushrooms (5-8)
- Water (2-4 cups)
- Onions (1/2 cup), chopped
- Carrots & celery (1/2 cup), chopped

Instructions

- In a saucepan, bring all ingredients to a boil, then reduce heat to low and enable to simmer for 10 minutes.

Chicken and Corn Chowder
Time: 40 Mins, Serves: 12, Skill: Easy

Ingredients

- Chicken breasts (8), boneless, diced
- Fresh thyme (6 tbsp), chopped
- Bacon (12 slices), low sodium
- Onions (2), chopped
- Chicken broth (7 cups), low sodium
- Turnips (4), diced & soaked
- Corn (5 cups)
- Unsweetened almond milk (4 cups)
- Black pepper (1/2 tsp)
- Green onions (8), chopped

Instructions

- Fry the bacon. Remove the bacon from the pan and place it on a plate to cool.
- Fry the onions in the bacon fat.
- After including the potatoes and broth, cover and simmer for 10 minutes.
- Add the chicken, corn, and thyme to the pot and cook until the chicken is thoroughly baked, (15 mins).
- Add the Mocha Mix to the broth, cook for 2 minutes.

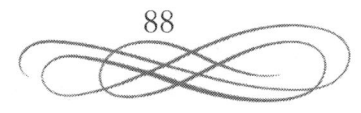

- Toss in the bacon, green onions, and season to taste with salt and pepper.

Simple Soup Base
Time: 1 hour, Serves: 4, Skill: Easy

Ingredients
- Paprika (1/4 tsp)
- Almond Flour (2 tbsp)
- Margarine or butter (2 tbsp)
- Almond Milk (2 cups)
- Dry mustard (1/4 tsp)
- Parsley, basil or any other herbs (1/2 tsp)

Instructions
- Mix margarine and almond flour in a microwave-safe dish.
- Microwave for 30 seconds on high, stir, then microwave for another 30 seconds on high.
- Add the spices and almond milk, and cook for another minute in the microwave.
- To thicken, microwave for another minute. Microwave for a further minute if the sauce isn't thick enough.
- It may be used in lieu of cream soups.

Texas-Style Chili
Time: 1 hour and 25 Mins, Serves: 6, Skill: Hard

Ingredients
- Onion (1 large)
- Fresh tomato sauce (1 cup)
- Water (2 cups)
- Green chili pepper (1/2 cup), finely chopped
- Red bell pepper (1), chopped
- Chili powder (2 tbsp)
- Lean ground beef (1 lb.)
- Garlic powder (1 tbsp)
- Cumin (1/4 tsp), ground
- Dried oregano (1/2 tsp)
- Dried thyme (1/2 tsp)
- Dried basil (1 tsp)
- Cajun seasoning (1/4 tsp)

Instructions
- In a big pot over medium heat, brown the beef.
- Add the onion and cook until it is soft, around 5 minutes.
- In a big mixing bowl, add 2 cups water, tomato sauce, bell pepper, green chilies, and spices.
- Bring to a simmer, then reduce to low heat and proceed to cook for around 1 hour.

Vibrant carrot soup
Time: 1 hour, Serves: 4, Skill: Easy

Ingredients
- Olive oil (1 tbsp)
- Ginger (2 tsp), grated
- Sweet onion (1/2), chopped
- Garlic (1 tsp), minced
- Carrots (3), chopped
- Water (4 cups)
- Coconut milk (1/2 cup)
- Turmeric (1 tsp), ground
- Cilantro (1 tbsp), chopped

Instructions
- Sauté the garlic, onion, and ginger in a saucepan of hot olive oil for 3 minutes over a high flame.
- Bring the turmeric, water, and carrots to a boil in a saucepan.
- Reduce the heat to low and proceed to cook for another 20 minutes.
- Put the soup mixture and vegetables into a blender and add the coconut milk to produce a smooth broth.
- Return the smooth soup mixture to the pan and heat until it has thickened to the consistency of a deep soup.
- Garnish with chopped cilantro.

Green Breakfast Soup
Time: 40 Mins, Serves: 2, Skill: Easy

Ingredients
- Vegetable broth (2 cups)
- Coriander (1 tsp), ground

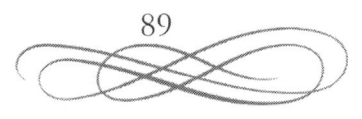

- Turmeric (1 tsp), Ground
- Cumin (1 tsp), ground
- Lettuce (1 cup)
- Black pepper, to taste

Instructions
- Mix the lettuce, coriander, turmeric, broth, and cumin in a food processor.
- Transfer the mixture to a skillet and cook over medium heat for 3 minutes.
- Season to taste with pepper and serve.

Vegetable Stew
Time: 50 Mins, Serves: 8, Skill: Easy

Ingredients
- Cayenne pepper (1 pinch)
- Garlic (1 tsp), chopped
- Red bell pepper (1), diced
- Tomatoes (2), chopped
- Coriander (1 tsp)
- Carrots (2), chopped
- Cumin (1/2 tsp)
- Zucchini (2), chopped
- Broccoli florets (2 cups)
- Onion (1), chopped
- Black pepper, to taste
- Olive oil (1 tsp)
- Cilantro (2 tbsp), chopped
- Vegetable stock (2 cups)

Instructions
- Heat the olive oil in a medium saucepan and sauté the garlic and onion.
- After adding the bell pepper, zucchini, and carrots, cook for another 5 minutes.
- Add the tomatoes, cumin, broccoli, cayenne pepper, and coriander.
- Reduce it to a low heat.
- Proceed to cook the vegetables for another 5 minutes.
- Garnish with cilantro and black pepper before serving.

Drink & Beverage Recipes

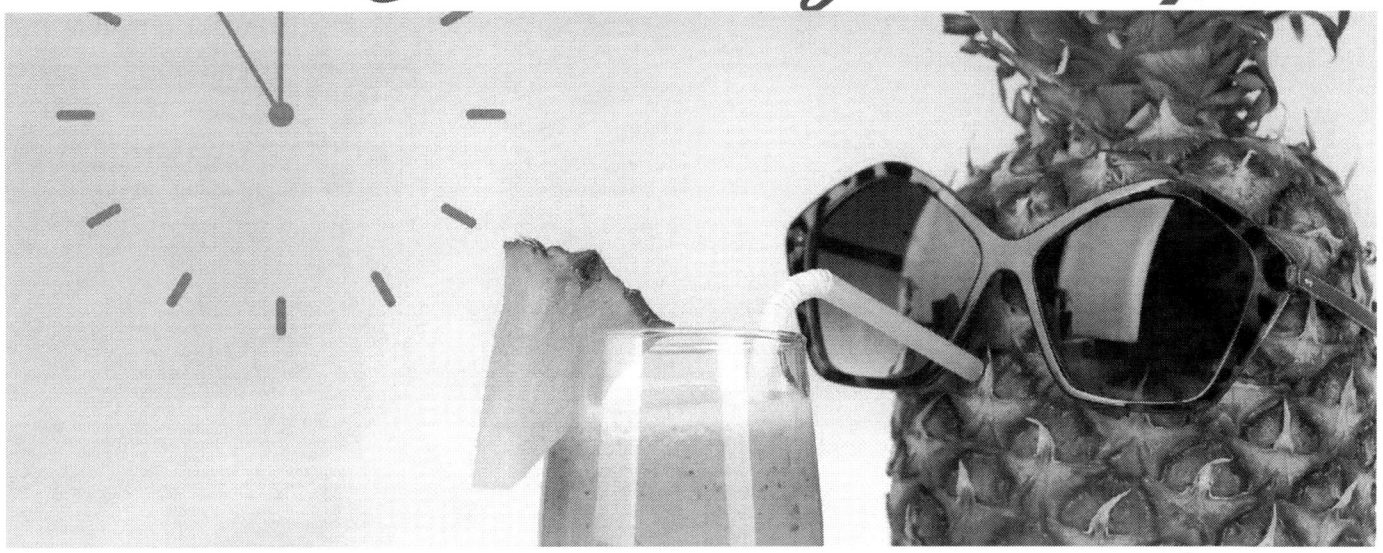

Refer to the end of the book for the conversion chart.

Apple Cup Cider
Time: 25 Mins, Serves: 4, Skill: Easy

Ingredients
- Cinnamon sticks (2)
- Whole cloves (1/2 tsp)
- Nutmeg (1 pinch)
- Allspice (1 tsp)
- Apple juice diluted with water (1 quart 100%)

Instructions
- In a large saucepan, heat the apple juice over medium-high heat.
- Add the remaining ingredients.
- Reduce to low heat after bringing to a low boil. Allow for a 10-minute "steeping" period.
- Pour the cider into a mug or thermos using the fine metal sieve.

Mixed Berry Protein Smoothie
Time: 12 Mins, Serves: 2, Skill: Easy

Ingredients
- Whey protein powder (2 scoops)
- Coldwater (4 oz.)
- Mixed berries (1 cup), fresh/frozen
- Ice cubes (2)
- Crystal Light (1 tsp), flavor enhancer drops (liquid, any berry flavor)

Instructions
- Combine all the ingredients in a blender until creamy.
- Load the protein powder into a broad mixing cup.

Lemon-Strawberry Punch
Time: 10 Mins, Serves: 1, Skill: Easy

Ingredients
- Sparkling water (1 l. bottle)
- Fresh Lemon juice (1 cup), add stevia (1 tbsp)
- Frozen strawberries (1 box 10 oz), in a light syrup, undrained and thawed

Instructions
- Whisk together the lemonade concentrate and 9 cans of water in a four-quart tub until well mixed.
- Fill a punch bowl halfway of lemonade. Strawberries may be combined in a number of ways.

- Apply the ice and ginger ale and whisk softly.

Vegan Hot Chocolate
Time: 15 Mins, Serves: 1, Skill: Easy

Ingredients
- Vanilla extract (1/2 tsp)
- Oat milk (1 cup)
- Cocoa powder (1 tbsp)
- Stevia (2 tsp)

Instructions
- Heat the milk in a small saucepan over medium-high heat.
- Combine the cocoa powder, vanilla extract, and stevia in a mixing cup.
- To mix, carefully whisk all the products together.
- Carry to a simmer before scalding (when bubbles emerge along the edges of the liquid in the pot).
- Extract it from the pan, put it into a mug, and serve.

Mexican Coconut Drink
Time: 25 Mins, Serves: 6, Skill: Easy

Ingredients
- Lime (4 slices)
- Water (2 cups)
- White rice (2 cups)
- Coconut water (2 cups), unsweetened
- Coconut milk (1 can), unsweetened
- Stevia (3 tsp)

Instructions
- Fill a saucepan halfway with water (2 cups), bring to a boil, and remove from heat as soon as possible.
- In a medium mixing bowl, combine the coconut water and rice; cover and set aside at room temperature for the night.
- Blend the rice and coconut water mixture until smooth the next day.
- Wrap a medium-sized dish in cheesecloth and secure it with a rubber band or twine.
- Using cheesecloth, strain the liquid from the rice puree.
- Pour the rice water into a strainer and discard the rice sediment.
- In a small saucepan, heat the coconut milk and stevia over low heat for 4 minutes, or until the sugar is fully dissolved.
- Pour the sweetened coconut mixture over the rice and chill before ready to serve.
- Serve with ice and lime juice, garnished with lime slices.

Lemonade
Time: 10 Mins, Serves: 2, Skill: Easy

Ingredients
- Ice cubes
- Water (2-1/2 cups)
- Stevia (1/4 cup)
- Lemon (1/2 tsp), finely shredded
- Fresh lemon or lime juice (1-1/4 cups)

Instructions
- Heat the water and sugar in a medium saucepan until the sugar has dissolved. Remove the pan from the heat and put it aside to cool for 20 minutes.
- In a large mixing cup, combine the lemon peel and juice. Allow to cool in a covered pitcher or pot. This can be held for up to three days.
- In a glass packed with ice, combine 3 oz. of base and 3 oz. of water to make a lemonade cocktail. Shake it up a little and serve.

Fruity Baked Tea
Time: 45 Mins, Serves: 1, Skill: Medium

Ingredients
- Apricots (1/2 cup), dried, diced
- Cloves (25 pieces)
- Star anise (4 pieces)
- Apple (1), diced
- Pear (1), diced
- Orange (1), diced
- Lemon (1), diced

- Peaches (1 cup), diced
- Berries (2 cups), blackberries, raspberries, blueberries, cherries, diced
- Powdered cinnamon (2 tsp)
- Brown sugar (2 tbsp)

Instructions

- Arrange all of the fruits in a baking bowl. Stir in all of the sugar and spices.
- Cover the bowl in aluminum foil to keep it dry. Bake for 40 minutes, stirring after 10 to 15 minutes.
- Remove the foil and bake for another 20 minutes to evaporate any juices and concentrate the taste.
- Extract the dish from the oven and automatically put the contents into four 8-ounce jars, or sixteen 2-ounce jars.
- Firmly seal the jars and encourage them to cool by standing on their lids with their bottoms up.
- Fill a medium saucepan halfway with water and bring to a boil. Boil for 15 minutes after inserting the bottoms of the jars.
- Remove the jars from the oven and put them aside to cool before placing them in the refrigerator.
- To serve, place 1 tablespoon of the mixture in a cup. Combine 8 oz. of boiling water in a glass and drink.

Strawberry Sesame Milkshake

Time: 16 Mins, Serves: 3, Skill: Easy

Ingredients

- Ice cubes (1 cup)
- Sesame seeds (1/2 tbsp), toasted
- Strawberries (1 lb.), halved
- Balsamic glaze (2 tbsp)
- Banana (1/2 small/50 grams), frozen, optional
- Coconut milk (1/2 cup)
- Tahini (2 tbsp)

Instructions

- Preheat the oven to 400 °F.
- In a mixing bowl, toss the strawberries with the balsamic glaze.
- Spread it out on a baking dish lined with parchment paper and set aside for 5 minutes.
- Cook for 10 minutes, then remove from the oven and flip the strawberries over to roast for another 10 minutes, or until softened.
- In a blender, combine the strawberries, coconut milk, tahini, pineapple, and ice and blend until smooth.
- Pour the smoothies into three glasses and top with toasted sesame seeds and a dry strawberry.

Rhubarb Tea

Time: 1 hour and 20 Mins, Serves: 8, Skill: Hard

Ingredients

- Mint, to garnish
- Rhubarb stalks (8)
- Water (8 cups)
- Stevia (3 cup)

Instructions

- Cut 8 rhubarb stalks into 3" sections, put in a pot of 8 cups water, bring to a boil, then reduce to low heat, and simmer for 1 hour.

Strain the drink, then apply about a third of a cup (or to taste) of stevia and put aside to cool.

Green Kiwi Smoothie

Time: 10 Mins, Serves: 1, Skill: Easy

Ingredients

- Water (1 cup)
- Stevia (1 tsp), optional
- Kiwi (1), peeled, chopped
- Kale (1/2 cup), fresh or frozen, stemmed & chopped
- Almonds (2 tbsp)
- Ice cubes (2)

Instructions

- Add all the ingredients in a blender and mix until smooth.

Dessert Recipes

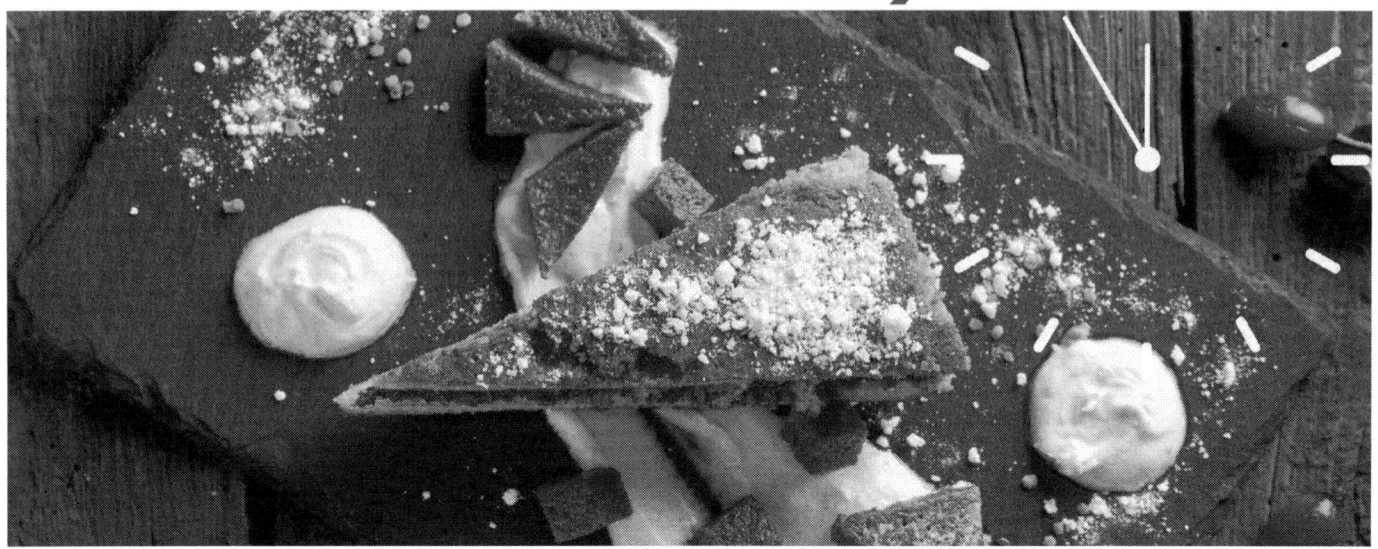

Refer to the end of the book for the conversion chart.

Sugarless Pecan and Raisin Cookies
Time: 55 Mins, Serves: 8, Skill: Medium

Ingredients
- Salt (1/2 tsp)
- Oil (1/4 cup)
- Egg (1)
- Pecans (1/2 cup)
- Cranberries (1/2 cup)
- Coconut Flour (3/4 cup)
- Baking powder (2 tsp)
- Cinnamon (1/2 tsp)
- Canned orange juice (3/4 cup), unsweetened
- Orange rind (1/2 tsp)

Instructions
- In a big mixing bowl, combine the flour, baking powder, salt, and cinnamon.
- Add and combine the remaining ingredients.
- Drop by the teaspoonful onto a baking sheet that hasn't been greased.
- Preheat oven to 375°F and bake for 15 to 20 minutes.

Crispy Butterscotch Cookies
Time: 40 Mins, Serves: 10, Skill: Easy

Ingredients
- Stevia (1/2 cup)
- Egg alternative (3 tbsp)
- Milk (1 tbsp)
- Vanilla extract (1 tsp)
- Margarine (1/2 cup)
- Ground flaxseed (1 cup)
- Butterscotch chips (1 cup), sugar free
- All-purpose flour (1 cup + 3 tbsp)
- Baking powder (1 tsp)
- Cinnamon (1/2 tsp), ground

Instructions
- Preheat the oven to 350 °F.
- In a mixing tub, cream together the stevia and butter.
- Add and whisk together the egg, chocolate, and milk. Using a blender, soften the mixture.
- In a mixing cup, combine the flour, cinnamon, and baking powder.
- Pour into the butter mixture and whisk well.

- Add in the butterscotch chips and ground flaxseed thoroughly.
- Drop teaspoons one at a time onto the prepared baking dish.
- Bake for 9–12 minutes, or until golden brown.
- Allow to cool on the baking sheet for 1 minute before switching to cooling racks.

Easy Spicy Angel Cake
Time: 40 Mins, Serves: 18, Skill: Easy

Ingredients
- Nutmeg (1/2 tsp), ground
- Ginger (1/4 tsp), ground
- Cloves (1/4 tsp), ground
- Angel food cake mix (1 pkg), sugar free
- Cinnamon (1 tsp), ground

Instructions
- In a bowl, combine all the ingredients.
- Begin cooking and baking as directed on the box.
- Set aside to cool.
- Cut each segment into one-inch pieces.
- Include a whipped topping and strawberry or pineapple to finish.

Apple Filled Crepes
Time: 30 Mins, Serves: 6, Skill: Easy

Ingredients
- Eggs (2)
- Stevia (1/2 cup)
- Almond flour (1 cup)
- Oil (1/4 cup)
- Milk (2 cups)
- Egg yolks (4)
- Apples (4 pieces)
- Brown sugar (1/4 cup)
- Cinnamon (1/2 tsp)
- Nutmeg (1/2 tsp)
- Butter (1 stick or 1/2 cup), unsalted

Instructions
- Whisk together the egg yolks, entire whites, stevia, flour, butter, and milk in a big mixing bowl until smooth.
- In a tiny nonstick pan, melt the oil over medium heat.
- Coat the bowl with nonstick cooking spray.
- Spoon 1 scoop of batter into the tub with a 2-ounce ladle or 1/4 cup, and roll the pan to evenly scatter the crepe batter on the bottom.
- Cook for 20 seconds, on one side, then flip and cook for another 10 seconds on the other. While we prepare the filling, set the crepes aside.
- Peel and core the apples, and cut them into 12 slices each.
- Steam the apples in a medium sauté pan.
- Eventually, apply the brown sugar to the melting butter.
- In a mixing dish, combine the cinnamon, apples, and nutmeg.
- Cook until the apples are tender but not soggy. Remove from the heat and set aside to cool.
- Fill each crepe's center with approximately two tablespoons of apple filling.

Chocolate Covered Strawberries
Time: 25 Mins, Serves: 2, Skill: Easy

Ingredients
- Corn syrup (1 tbsp), sugar free
- Margarine (5 tbsp)
- Strawberries (1 qtr.)
- Chocolate chips (1/2 cup), semi-sweet

Instructions
- Over a low flame, melt the first three ingredients.
- Blend until fully smooth.
- Switch off the heat and cover the pan with water.
- Put strawberries on waxed paper after dipping them in chocolate.

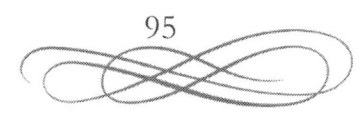

- Place the food in the fridge to cool before serving.

Apple Oat Shake
Time: 30 Mins, Serves: 4, Skill: Easy

Ingredients
- Wheat germ (1 tbsp)
- Vanilla extract (1 1/2 tsp)
- Frozen apple (1/2 pieces), cut into chunks
- Oatmeal (1/2 cup), cooked, chilled
- Skim milk (2/3 cup)
- Stevia (2 tbsp)

Instructions
- Blend the oatmeal for a couple minutes in a blender.
- In a large mixing cup, whisk together the milk, vanilla, stevia, wheat germ, and half of the apple mixture.
- Blend until the mixture has reached a creamy, dense consistency.

Molten Mint Chocolate Brownies
Time: 40 Mins, Serves: 8, Skill: Easy

Ingredients
- Andes mint chocolates (12 pieces), sugar free
- Optional garnish: cocoa powder, powdered sugar, fresh mint springs,
- Betty Crocker brownie mix (1 box), sugar free

Instructions
- Preheat the oven to 350°F and follow the product instructions for cooking the brownie mix.
- In a 12-cup muffin pan that has been lined or lightly oiled, flour the bottom sheet. Bake for 25 minutes after putting the brownie mix in the pans.
- After placing one slice of mint candy in the middle, bake for an additional 5 minutes. Remove the brownies from the oven and place them on a cooling rack to cool. Allow for 5–10 minutes of cooling before serving.

Blueberry Whipped Pie
Time: 1 hour and 30 Mins, Serves: 9, Skill: Medium

Ingredients
- Graham cracker crumbs (2 cups)
- Cinnamon (1 tsp)
- Monk fruit (1/4 cup)
- Lemon juice (2 tsp)
- Vanilla extract (1 tsp)
- Whipped cream (8 oz. tub), non-dairy
- Blueberries (3 cups)
- Butter (1/2 cup), melted, unsalted
- Cream cheese (8 oz.), softened

Instructions
- Preheat oven to 375°F.
- Put the cinnamon sticks, graham cracker crumbs, monk fruit, and melted butter in a medium mixing cup.
- To make a crust, thinly scatter the mixture in the bottom of a 9-inch circular or square baking dish.
- After baking, allow for 7 minutes of cooking time.
- In a big mixing tub, using a hand processor, smooth out the melted cream cheese.
- In a mixing cup, combine the vanilla and lemon juice.
- Before applying the blueberries, fold in the whipped topping softly.
- Cover the whole surface with the paste.
- After covering, place in the refrigerator for at least 1 hour.

Yellow Cake
Time: 1 hour and 25 Mins, Serves: 8, Skill: Medium

Ingredients
- Stevia (2/3 cup)
- Water (1/2 cup)
- Egg (1)
- Vanilla (1/2 tsp)
- Master Mix (1 1/2 cups)

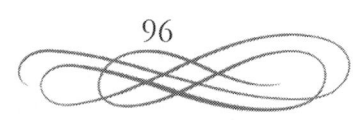

Instructions
- Preheat the oven to 375 °F.
- For Master Mix, follow the steps outlined.
- Add some stevia to the mixture.
- In a separate dish, whisk together the egg, water, and vanilla extract.
- Beat for 2 minutes after adding half of the solvent to the mixture.
- Pour in the remaining liquid and continue to beat for 2 minutes.
- Bake for 25 minutes in a tray lined with wax paper.
- One 8-inch layer is made for this recipe.

Tropical Fruit Salad with Basil Lime Syrup

Time: 1 hour and 10 Mins, Serves: 10, Skill: Medium

Ingredients
- Strawberries (1 1/2 cup), sliced
- Mango (1 cup), cubed
- Water (1/4 cup)
- Stevia (1/4 cup)
- Lime zest (1 1/2 tsp)
- Packed basil leaves (1/4 cup)

Instructions
- Bring water to a boil in a small frying pan and stir in stevia.
- Boil and cook until completely dissolved.
- Take the pan off the heat and stir in the lime zest and basil.
- In a large mixing cup, combine the fruits while the syrup cools.
- Soak the cheesecloth or strainer in the syrup to remove the solids.
- Serve as a side dish of fruits or as a snack.

Conversion Chart

UK-US

Spoons, Cup & Liquid

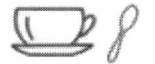 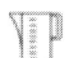

Spoons & Cups	ml
¼ tsp	1.25 ml
½ tsp	2.5 ml
1 tsp	5 ml
1 tbsp	15 ml
¼ cup	60 ml
1/3 cup	80 ml
½ cup	125 ml
1 cup	250 ml

Temperature

Gas Mark	°C	°F
1	140 °C	275 °F
2	150 °C	300 °F
3	170 °C	325 °F
4	180 °C	350 °F
5	190 °C	375 °F
6	200 °C	400 °F
7	220 °C	425 °F
8	230 °C	450 °F
9	240 °C	475 °F

American Cups to Grams

Ingredients	Grams	Ingredients	Grams
1 cup butter	225g	1 cup syrup	350g
1 cup flour	125g	1 cup rice (uncooked)	200g
1 cup white sugar	225g	1 cup brown sugar	200g

28-Days Meal Plan

In this meal plan, we consider 3 main meals for each day. They can be considered breakfast, lunch, and dinner, or even in another way, depending on your chosen Intermittent Fasting plan.

In addition to these 3 main meals, you can add a snack: a fruit, a protein bar, a Greek yogurt, mixed nuts, and anything else that does not contain carbohydrates. You can also refer to the Snacks & Side Recipes chapter.

For the fasting type 5:2, in the 2 days of low calories, you can eat just one of the meals of the food plan, plus a salad or snack of your choice from the recipes.

WEEK 1

page

Monday
Meal 1: Mexican Egg & Tortilla Skillet — 60
Meal 2: Baked Salmon
Meal 3: Curry Chicken — 68

Tuesday
Meal 1: Homemade Muesli
Meal 2: Spiced Pepitas
Meal 3: Coconut Fish Dream

Wednesday
Meal 1: Cheesesteak Quiche
Meal 2: Spanish Paella
Meal 3: Quick Mushroom Broth

Thursday
Meal 1: Cherry Overnight Oats
Meal 2: Chicken Veronique
Meal 3: Fajitas

Friday
Meal 1: Egg Sandwich
Meal 2: Chicken Waldorf Salad
Meal 3: Beef Curry

Saturday
Meal 1: Easy-baked pears
Meal 2: Fiesta Lime Tacos
Meal 3: Crab Cakes

Sunday
Meal 1: Burritos with Eggs and Mexican Sausage
Meal 2: Seasoned Pork Chops
Meal 3: Grilled Trout
Dessert: Yellow Cake

WEEK 2

Monday
Meal 1: Crepes with passion fruit
Meal 2: Shrimp Fajitas
Meal 3: Jamaican Beef Patties
Tuesday
Meal 1: Cherry Overnight Oats
Meal 2: Tortilla Beef Rollups
Meal 3: Basic Chicken Loaf
Wednesday
Meal 1: Creamy Fruit Salad
Meal 2: Barley-Rice Pilaf
Meal 3: Easy Beef Burgers
Thursday
Meal 1: Cheesesteak Quiche
Meal 2: Beef Curry
Meal 3: Broiled Garlic Shrimp
Friday
Meal 1: Fruity Chicken Salad
Meal 2: Simple Puerto Rican Sofrito
Meal 3: Tortilla Beef Rollups
Saturday
Meal 1: Egg Sandwich
Meal 2: Turkey Salad
Meal 3: Seafood Croquettes
Sunday
Meal 1: Oriental Egg Rolls
Meal 2: Parsley Burger
Meal 3: Salmon Salad
Dessert: Apple Oat Shake

WEEK 3

Monday
Meal 1: Cheesesteak Quiche
Meal 2: Seasoned Pork Chops
Meal 3: Chicken Veronique
Tuesday
Meal 1: Fresh Fruit Compote
Meal 2: Salisbury Steak
Meal 3: Chili Rice with Beef
Wednesday
Meal 1: Cherry Overnight Oats
Meal 2: Beef Casserole
Meal 3: Stir Fry Meal
Thursday
Meal 1: Egg Sandwich
Meal 2: Tortilla Beef Rollups
Meal 3: Wild Rice Salad
Friday
Meal 1: Mexican Egg & Tortilla Skillet
Meal 2: Baked Salmon
Meal 3: Spiced Pepitas
Saturday
Meal 1: Homemade Muesli
Meal 2: Crab Cakes
Meal 3: Easy Chicken and Pasta Dinner
Sunday
Meal 1: Burritos with Eggs and Mexican Sausage
Meal 2: Hawaiian-Style Slow-Cooked Beef
Meal 3: Coconut Fish Dream
Dessert: Chocolate Covered Strawberries

WEEK 4

Monday
Meal 1: Crepes with passion fruit
Meal 2: Turkey Salad
Meal 3: Tortilla Beef Rollups

Tuesday
Meal 1: Cherry Overnight Oats
Meal 2: Tortilla Beef Rollups
Meal 3: Seafood Croquettes

Wednesday
Meal 1: Homemade Muesli
Meal 2: Shrimp Fajitas
Meal 3: Thai Chicken Soup

Thursday
Meal 1: Deviled Eggs
Meal 2: Jamaican Beef Patties
Meal 3: Chicken and Corn Chowder

Friday
Meal 1: Creamy Fruit Salad
Meal 2: Curry Chicken
Meal 3: Wild Rice Soup

Saturday
Meal 1: Fruity Chicken Salad
Meal 2: Parsley Burger
Meal 3: Minestrone Soup

Sunday
Meal 1: Egg Sandwich
Meal 2: Beef Curry
Meal 3: Broiled Garlic Shrimp
Dessert: Apple Filled Crepes

A Free Gift for You

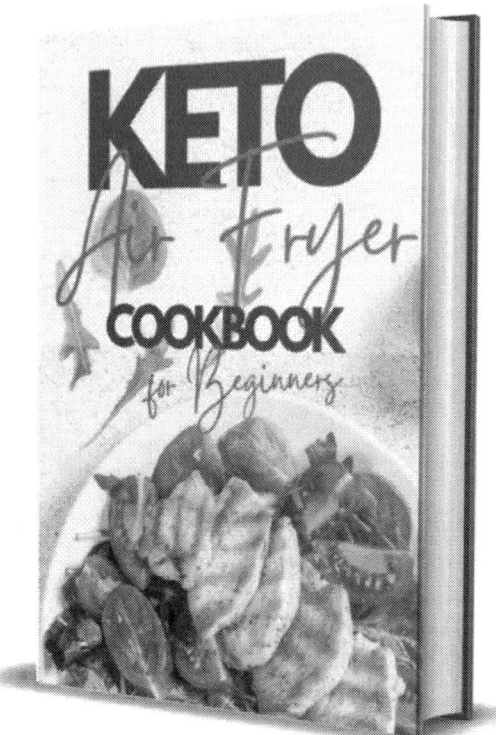

This book has a website containing some **helpful resources** for Intermittent Fasting.

On the website, you will find the following:

- **A fantastic Keto Air Fryer Cookbook for Beginners** written by a very close friend of mine, Emily Finner. **Air-fried foods contain up to 80% less fat** in comparison to deep-fried foods. Air frying is revolutionary for cooking **tasty but healthy dishes** that you can eat during your eating windows.
- **Links to the mobile apps** mentioned in the book and others will come in the future. Apps are an easy way **to monitor your Intermittent Fasting.**
- **Videos execution of the home exercises** described in the book.

Visit the website and discover all the free resources I have designed for you.

Follow this link
wiseapublishing.com/ifover50/bonus

or scan the QR code

Conclusion

You have been given all the tools you might need to learn all there is to know about Intermittent Fasting over the age of 50. Now it is all up to you. You should know by now how valuable this feeding plan can be for you, especially as you grow older. It is not just about shedding some extra pounds or boosting your metabolism. It is also about increasing your lifespan, making you feel healthier and more content about things that happen every day. It is a once-in-a-lifetime opportunity to reset your body and start over. Don't you want this transformation?

It is just the beginning of the journey. You might feel anxious, overwhelmed by information, and eager to see what lies ahead. Don't be in a hurry. Let the journey take you where you want to be, offering you amazing benefits. After all, it is a work in progress. As you dive deeper, you realize more details about Intermittent Fasting. You will discover more details about how your body works and responds to different situations. Over time, you will understand which foods are good for you and which ones you should omit from your diet plan. And as you see that transformation slowly taking place, your determination strengthens. Learning to interpret the signs and allow your body to heal itself is fascinating.

Do not just choose to fast without first reading all about it. This would be a disaster. You should know by now your body is complex, with various layers needing exploration. Give yourself time to study and realize what is best for you in the long run. Turn to science whenever you are experiencing even the slightest sliver of doubt. Do not let it simmer, as it will become an even more important issue. Clear the air, leave nothing unanswered, and ease yourself into Intermittent Fasting when ready.

I hope this book has been an inspirational guide as you embark on your journey, which is just beginning. I wish you all the best and eagerly anticipate the revolutionary changes set to unfold in your life. Witnessing the transformation in people who have embraced Intermittent Fasting is truly exhilarating. They emerge radiant, completely renewed, and brimming with hope for the future.

If you found value in this book, I kindly ask you to write a review to help other women discover it and embark on their own transformative journeys. Your insights and experiences can be a guiding light for many.

You can email me at
amberlane@wiseapublishing.com

Manufactured by Amazon.ca
Bolton, ON